MW01034793

Medical Marijuana and CBD

Medical Marijuana
and CBD

A Physician's Guide for Patients

Matthew Mintz, MD, FACP

© 2020 by Matthew Mintz

All rights reserved. This book or any portion thereof may not be reproduced or used in any manner whatsoever without the express written permission of the publisher except for the use of brief quotations in a book review.

ISBN: 978-1-7351554-0-1

Contents

Foreword

You can find almost anything on the internet—or so I thought. When I first starting certifying patients for medical cannabis and needed to learn more, I first went to the typical medical resources to which I turn: major journal articles (like *The New England Journal of Medicine*) as well as websites designed for physicians only that aggregate some of this information (such as Up to Date). Not surprisingly, there was little to no information about medical cannabis, so like most patients, I turned to the internet. The internet has previously helped me learn things on my own in critical situations (changing a sink faucet, replacing the air filter on my car, et cetera), so I assumed that learning about medical cannabis would be no different. While there was plenty of information regarding medical marijuana, there was very little practical information about how to use medical marijuana for patients with specific conditions. There was a lot of information about medical marijuana being effective (some even had journal references). There was some basic information about medical marijuana, some of which was useful, such as describing different cannabis strains and terpenes, and some was not so useful (at least from a physician or patient standpoint), such as how to grow medical cannabis or how to advocate for the legalization of cannabis. Since the internet failed me, I next went to Amazon to see if perhaps there was a book that might explain all of this, but while there were several books containing similar information, I could not find one book written by a physician for patients or other physicians that explained exactly how to use medical cannabis for a specific medical condition. While this was frustrating as a physician, I could not imagine how difficult this must be for an ill patient seeking information. This left me no choice but to spend countless hours searching for information and educating myself. Since the type of book that I was looking for appeared not to exist, I also decided I would write one.

The information and opinions in this book are based on the existing research I was able to find, information from courses I have taken, speaking to a number of experts in the area of medical cannabis, and most importantly, the successes and failures from over a thousand patients I have certified for medical cannabis in Maryland and the District of Columbia. While this book discusses the science of medical cannabis (there is an entire chapter on research), this is not meant to be a scientific or medical book—though I do hope the book contains enough scientific information to convince patients and clinicians that the science behind medical cannabis is sound. This book also will not focus on topics that I don't believe are of significant importance to ill medical patients or their doctors, such as how to grow cannabis, how to make your own medical cannabis products, or how to advocate for the legalization of medical cannabis. Rather, my hope is that this books will provide the information needed for a patient who has decided to try medical cannabis but doesn't know what to do next, as well as for the patient who is considering medical cannabis for their condition but is not sure if medical cannabis is right for them.

Introduction

My Journey with Medical Marijuana

I never imagined that I would become a staunch advocate for the use of medical marijuana. I was a pretty straight and narrow teenager and young adult, never having even tried drugs, including marijuana. We never learned about medical marijuana in medical school. What we did learn about marijuana was that it was a Schedule I drug, meaning it was illegal, was addictive, and had no real benefit. Even later as a practicing physician, I had heard about some use of marijuana to relieve pain and suffering in cancer patients. While I saw no problem with this as a last resort, given that there was very limited data (at least in the journals that I read), it did not seem like something that would be relevant for many of my patients. I was even aware of some of the medicinal properties of THC. THC had been around since the late 1980s as a prescription drug. I remember prescribing Marinol (dronabinol) during my residency for hospitalized patients with severe nausea (usually as a side effect from chemotherapy) when other more common medications were not working. For the few patients I prescribed this medication for, I was not that impressed with the results. Having practiced in the District of Columbia for most of my medical career, I was aware the medical marijuana would eventually be legal in the area where I practiced. However, I had heard that many of the logistics of the dispensaries had yet to be worked out, and it was my impression that it would be years before medical marijuana might be something I could actually use for patients.

However, all of this changed when I left my job as full-time faculty at the George Washington University School of Medicine, where I had been teaching and seeing patients for twenty years. For a variety of reasons, I decided to open my own practice in Bethesda, Maryland, in July 2017. Like any new medical practice, it takes some time to get new patients. Most practices take two to three years to get up and running. Thus, the fall of 2017 was pretty slow for me. However, in December 2017, I learned that a medical marijuana dispensary was opening in my medical office building. Curious, I met with the owners, who told me a bit more about the benefits of medical cannabis. They also informed me that very few physicians were actually signed up with the state of Maryland to certify patients for medical marijuana. In fact, many of the providers who had registered to certify patients were not actually physicians but were podiatrists, dentists, or nurse practitioners. In addition, most of the clinics that advertised they were certifying patients for medical marijuana were set up as cash businesses that exclusively certified patients without using physicians or providing regular medical care. I was intrigued, so I investigated medical marijuana a little bit more. While the traditional sources of medical information that I typically use to update myself on medical topics had little regarding evidence behind the use of medical marijuana, the internet had a ton of information about the benefits, and possibly more importantly, the safety of medical marijuana. Thus, I decided that certifying patients for medical marijuana might be a good way to help patients while my practice slowly grew.

I will admit that I initially had some reservations about certifying patients for medical marijuana. I worried that patients I would see might simply be looking for an excuse to use recreational marijuana legally. However, it became clear fairly quickly that this simply was not the case. My office in Bethesda, Maryland, is just outside the District of Columbia, where recreational marijuana was now legal. Thus, people in my area who just want to get pot legally go to our nation's capital to get it. It is much easier to get, and significantly less expensive than medically regulated cannabis. Likely because of this fact, and perhaps because I was one of the only physicians in my area to publicly declare that I would be certifying patients for medical marijuana as part of my regular medical practice, the patients who came to see me turned out to be quite sick. Some of the first few patients I saw included a woman with metastatic breast cancer who had severe nausea from her chemotherapy, a young adult man with very severe anxiety who had tried every prescription medication imaginable with no relief, and a middle-aged woman with severe and debilitating chronic pain from severe arthritis who was now addicted to opioid pain relievers and desperate for an alternative to these dangerous medications. Some of the initial patients who came to see me had tried just about everything to treat their conditions, and either nothing worked, or they had severe side effects from their prescription medications and were interested in medical marijuana as a last resort. Others had tried recreational marijuana and found it to be the only thing that helped their chronic conditions and came to me for certification so they could obtain the one thing that worked for them safely and legally. After seeing so many of these types of patients, I was convinced more than ever that my decision to certify patients for medical marijuana was the right thing to do.

Since that time, I have researched and learned as much as I can about medical marijuana, and I continue to strive to find the most up-to-date information. In addition, I have now had the privilege of certifying over a thousand patients for medical cannabis and have learned from their experiences, including responses to various treatment options. While initially skeptical, I have been extremely impressed with the results of medical cannabis as a therapeutic agent. While research is still very limited due to the fact that marijuana is federally illegal and there are no large pharmaceutical companies funding research, my experience has been consistent with the research that does exist, showing medical cannabis to be effective for a variety of conditions including chronic pain, anxiety, migraine, insomnia, and nausea.

Medicinal cannabis (the more clinically appropriate term for medical marijuana) is very different from recreational pot. Recreational pot is used for social purposes, to get "stoned" or "high." Medical cannabis is meant to be used as a medicine. While the marijuana plant—known as bud, herb, or flower—can be legally obtained for smoking in thirty-three states, such as Maryland, where I practice, and the District of Columbia, I don't recommend smoking cannabis, as there are multiple formulations such as pills, liquids, tincture, creams, transdermal, and vape that can be used and dosed more like a medication. In addition, medical cannabis is not just one therapy. There is a large variety of marijuana plant strains that can be used to treat different medical conditions. Some are strains are good for pain, some are good for sleep, and some can even make you feel more alert during this day. Thus, when using marijuana as a medicine, we can recommend specific compounds that will alleviate suffering without causing a "high." Based on my experience, I am now recommending medical cannabis to patients in my regular practice who had not previously considered this.

Unfortunately, most of my physician colleagues are reluctant to recommend medical cannabis. In fact, one of my first cancer patients stated that their oncologist wouldn't even discuss medical cannabis with her in regard to treating her symptoms. (This patient was actually the one who recommend I should speak to other doctors in the area to tell them about the benefits of medical cannabis and got me started on this pathway of sharing information with patients and colleagues.) One reason for physician reluctance is that while there is certainly research available, it generally is not composed of the large, randomized clinical trials that we physicians are used to when it comes to prescribing medications. Because of this lack of research, mostly due to current restrictive federal regulations, there is little guidance on which strains are best for which conditions, as well as the best formulations and doses for a given condition. In many cases, it is the patient care specialist at the dispensary (known as a "bud tender") that is providing this type of information to patients, which makes doctors very uncomfortable. This lack of information for patients and doctors is one of the main reasons I have written this book. Finally, even though most medical marijuana laws are written in a very physician-friendly way, and there is legal precedent protecting physicians who recommend marijuana for patients in a state where it is legal, because marijuana is federally illegal, many physicians have legal concerns about recommending medical cannabis, as well as concerns about malpractice.

However, when physicians recommend any treatment, we always think in terms of two things: safety and efficacy. *Safety* refers to whether a treatment will have side effects or harm the patient. *Efficacy* refers to how well a treatment actually works. Every decision we make in medical therapy is a balance of safety and efficacy of a given treatment, along with the risks and benefits of not taking that treatment. For example, while there is a certain risk for any surgical procedure, an appendectomy has a relatively low risk of complications and is very effective at removing an infected appendix, and not removing an infected appendix could be life threatening. In these terms, I would argue that medical marijuana is not only safe and effective for a variety of conditions, but it is also at least as effective and certainly safer than many of the prescription medications that we use to treat conditions like anxiety, pain, and insomnia. Even ibuprofen, which is over-the-counter, can cause gastrointestinal bleeding and kidney failure. Tylenol is a leading cause of liver failure in the United States. While I believe there are many patients who can benefit from medical cannabis, because of its excellent safety and efficacy profile, there are two patient groups in particular for whom I think physicians need to start considering medical marijuana as part of regular treatment: patients on opioid pain medications and the elderly.

We are in the midst of an opioid crisis, where over one hundred people are dying every day from opioid-related overdoses. There are multiple studies showing that patients who use medical cannabis can lower their narcotic doses, and epidemiologic data showing that in states that have legalized medical marijuana, doctors write one thousand fewer pain medication prescriptions per physician, and these states have significantly lower death rates from opioids. Finally, while narcotic medications are prescribed legally and marijuana is still federally illegal, it should be noted that no one has ever died from use of cannabis of any kind.

Most of the regular patients in my new practice have come from doctors who have recently retired. Because of this, the patients in my new practice tend to be slightly older than patients I was seeing at the medical school. While I am not a board-certified geriatrician, it is not a stretch to say that I have a significant number of geriatric patients in my new practice. Geriatric patients are usually taking multiple medications to treat a variety of conditions, all of which have side effects and can interact with each other. In addition to common ailments such as high blood pressure and high cholesterol, geriatric patients often take prescriptions for pain, insomnia, and anxiety. Medical cannabis is a natural, nonaddictive product that is very effective at treating all of these conditions, with few to no side effects, and little to any interactions with most prescription medications.

In addition to limited research, which may take a very long time to correct in our current political environment, stigma remains a major barrier to the appropriate use of medical cannabis. The marijuana plant has been used as a medicine for thousands of years. Many of the prescription medications we use today to treat conditions like pain, heart disease, and emphysema are derived from plants. Medical cannabis is a plant-based product that acts on receptors in the human body with a variety of therapeutic benefits. Given its excellent safety and efficacy compared to other treatments, especially for patients with chronic pain on narcotic medications and older patients having issues with sleep, anxiety, and/or pain, physicians and patients need to look beyond the recreational use marijuana and consider medical marijuana as a mainstream treatment for a variety of conditions.

Thus, the purpose of this book is to destigmatize the use of medical cannabis and provide evidence-based information to help patients who may benefit from this treatment (as well as clinicians who are looking for a concise, evidence-based resource). This book also contains an entire section on CBD, as CBD is an important component of treating patients when using cannabis, and hemp-based CBD is readily available (and legal) everywhere in the United States. In addition to reviewing how medical cannabis and CBD works, as well as the evidence behind its use, one thing unique to this book is that I will guide you through the process of getting medical cannabis and CBD, along with instructions on how to treat your specific condition. The recommendations in this book are gathered from my own research, interviews with cannabis experts, and the experience I have had in making recommendations to my patients. There are several books and internet sites that may describe medical marijuana or discuss some of the properties of the various strains. However, unlike anything that I have found on the internet (or in other published books), in this book I will give you detailed instructions about which products to take, how to use them, and how to adjust dosages for specific medical conditions. The last section contains several chapters; each one is for a common disease that can be effectively treated with medical cannabis, the content of which is derived from instructions I have given my own patients. My hope is that in the near future, regulations will change, more data will be available on the best methods to take medical cannabis for specific diseases, stigma will decrease, and eventually most doctors will be as comfortable recommending and educating patients on medical cannabis as they are with cholesterol-lowering medications. Until that time, I am hopeful that this book will empower the many patients interested in the benefits of medical cannabis and CBD, as well as the doctors who treat these patients.

Part A:

Medical Marijuana 101

Chapter 1:

The History of Medical Marijuana

What Is Medical Marijuana?

Marijuana is a plant that has been used as a medicine for thousands of years. In fact, many of the medicines we use today to treat conditions like emphysema, heart disease, and pain are derived from plants. Digoxin is derived from the plant *Digitalis purpurea*, or foxglove, and has been used for decades for the management of congestive heart failure. Atropine-based medicines, which are used for everything from stomach cramps, to emphysema, to runny noses, come from the plant *Atropa belladonna*, or nightshade. Even aspirin was originally derived from *Salix alba*, or the willow tree. More recently, we have the medication Taxol, which is commonly used to treat certain cancers, including breast cancer. It is derived from the bark of the Pacific yew tree, or *Taxis brevifolia*. Finally, both the strong painkillers known as narcotics, as well as drugs of abuse like heroin, are opioids that are given that name because they are derived from *Papaver somniferum*, or opium poppy. Because of the stigma and legal issues surrounding medical marijuana, it is important to point out that similar to the opioids, marijuana is a plant that is legally used to make medications that can help many people, and that the exact same plant can also be used to make illegal recreational drugs. It is ironic that prescription opioids are widely accepted by the public and medical community, but the ability of marijuana to be used as both a medicine and recreational drug is not, especially since while narcotics have and can been very beneficial, they are responsible to a huge opioid epidemic that has killed thousands of patients. Marijuana, used medicinally or recreationally, has never killed anyone.

Before continuing, it is important to discuss some botany and no-menclature. Marijuana is a plant known by the scientific name *cannabis*. *Cannabis* refers to a genus of plants that has three species: *indica*, *sativa*, and *ruderalis*. There is some debate how distinct these species really are, and some refer to *Cannabis sativa* as the proper name for all variations. While policies around the medicinal use of cannabis often use the term "marijuana" (e.g., getting my "medical marijuana card" and going to a "medical marijuana dispensary"), the term *marijuana* is usually associated with recreational use. Since cannabis is a scientific name, and medicine is a science, I believe it is more appropriate to use the term "cannabis" when discussing medicinal uses of marijuana. Thus, moving forward, I will use the term "medical cannabis" when discussing medical uses for this plant.

While the marijuana plant can be smoked and used as a recreational drug, medical cannabis is a natural treatment for a variety of medical conditions; when used correctly it will not get patients "high," and it does not have to be smoked. Medical cannabis comes in a variety of formulations, including pills, liquids, tinctures, and even topical creams. In thirty-three states and the District of Columbia, medical cannabis has been legally authorized to treat a number of specific conditions such as nausea, glaucoma, and seizures (this list varies by state). It can also be very useful in a variety of common conditions such as anxiety, insomnia, and chronic pain. Unlike some prescription medications, medical cannabis is safe, nonaddictive, and has few to no side effects or interactions with other medications. Many patients whom I have certified for medical cannabis decide to use it when their prescription medicines aren't working or are causing too many side effects.

Medical Cannabis in Early Times
While it is unclear when humans first started using marijuana as a medicine, or for recreational use, for that matter, medicinal text from China dating back several centuries BC report the use of the cannabis plant in medicine. Ayurvedic medicine is also a centuries-old form of

Indian medicine in which food and plants are commonly prescribed, and medical cannabis has been found in centuries-old Ayurvedic text as well. Even in Greek and Roman times, the use of medical cannabis has been described by some of our earliest physicians, such as Galen.

Medical Cannabis in the Nineteenth and Twentieth Centuries

One of the first reports of medical marijuana being used by "modern science" was in a paper published by Dr. William O'Shaughnessy in 1839 titled "Extract from a Memoir on the Preparations of the Indian Hemp, or Gunjah."[1] Dr. O'Shaughnessy described the benefits of cannabis being used in India when he traveled there.

By the midnineteenth century into the early twentieth century, extracts from the cannabis plant were incorporated into elixirs and other tonics to treat a variety of conditions. Drug companies such as Parke Davis, Lilly, and Wyeth had incorporated cannabis extracts into their popular products. Thus, cannabis was one of the first modern medicines in Europe and in the United States, predating antibiotics.

However, the popular use of marijuana, both recreationally and medicinally, decreased substantially in the midtwentieth century with the passage of the Marihuana Tax Act of 1937. Similar to the prohibition of alcohol that preceded it, there were concerns in some parts of society that marijuana use was sinful and dangerous, exemplified in the 1936 film *Refer Madness*. In addition to antimarijuana advocacy at the time, the 1937 Tax Act made it financially difficult for manufacturers to produce medicinal products containing cannabis, and thus the 1937 Tax Act essentially halted the progression of cannabis as a medicine for decades.

It was not until the 1960s that the medical benefits of cannabis were rediscovered in the United States. Frequent marijuana and other recreational drug use by "hippies" led to reports of medicinal benefits in a variety of conditions. It was reported that the severe nausea caused by the earliest and most caustic chemotherapeutic agents could be somewhat mitigated by smoking marijuana.

Around this same time, the science behind cannabis was just starting to emerge. Pioneer Israeli researcher Dr. Raphael Mechoulam was the first to identify and isolate delta-9 tetrahydrocannabinol, or THC, as one of the main active ingredients of marijuana in 1964.[2] While the increased use of marijuana in the '60s, reports of medicinal benefits, and research such as Dr. Mechoulam's should have propelled the use of medical cannabis along similar pathways of other fantastic new medicines in the 1970s and '80s, it was once again federal legislation that halted further progress.

Federal regulations and the FDA were still in their infancy in the '70s, and it was the passage of the Controlled Substances Act of 1970[3] that sealed the fate of medical marijuana. The Controlled Substances Act sought to more carefully regulate medicines that could be useful but also highly addictive or dangerous. They developed a scheduling system of various classes of drugs with regulations regarding who could prescribe and dispense these medications. For example, currently, controlled substances like opioids cannot be called into pharmacies like other medications, but rather can only be filled on a handwritten prescription or specially encrypted electronic prescription, and only by certain types of doctors. The controlled substance act defines a Schedule I drug as a drug or medication that is highly addictive with no medicinal value. Despite the existing data at that time, marijuana was classified as a Schedule I drug, making it essentially illegal. Given the increased interest and research in medical marijuana by doctors and patients, a scientific commission was convened in 1972 and recommended that marijuana be rescheduled as a Schedule II drug. Despite that recommendation, under President Nixon—who saw the criminalization of cannabis as a way to stall antiwar protestors—Attorney General John Mitchell (who later resigned to run Nixon's reelection campaign and eventually spent time in jail for his role in the Watergate scandal) maintained cannabis as a Schedule I in 1972, and it remains so to this day.[4] Because medical cannabis is federally illegal, in addition to some patients not being able to use it, scientists in the United States cannot perform the needed research on medical cannabis. Research restrictions are not just limited to federal institutions like the National Institutes of Health (NIH), but any major research institution, like a medical school, which relies on federal funding for its other research initiatives, will simply not perform cannabis research for fear of losing such funding.

While the Controlled Substances Act of 1970 curtailed the research and use of medical cannabis that had been reignited in the 1960s, another resurgence occurred in the 1990s with the AIDS epidemic. Wasting syndromes occurred with patients infected with HIV, and marijuana started to be used to stimulate appetite and help with weight gain. Given limited treatment options for HIV at the time, and a bureaucracy in the FDA that delayed getting patients the medications they so desperately needed, AIDS activists began to fight for access to treatments. This included staging protests, as well as use of buyers' clubs, where paying members could get illegal medications for free, with cannabis being used as one of these medicines. In 1996, California Proposition 215 was passed, essentially legalizing medical marijuana in the state of California. The law stated that California patients could possess and cultivate marijuana for any illness for which medical cannabis was expected to provide some relief. The legalization of medical cannabis in the state of California finally cracked open the gates to its use today. Medical cannabis is now legal in thirty-three states and the District of Columbia. In addition, we now have not only reports of successful use, but also actual research into the benefits of cannabis for a variety of conditions, including nausea, glaucoma, chronic pain, muscle spasms, and post-traumatic stress disorder, to name a few.

Finally, in addition to using nature's cannabis as a medicine, the pharmaceutical industry became interested in the medicinal uses of cannabis and its components. Building on the research of Dr. Mechoulam, drug companies were able to synthesize THC, and in 1986, Marinol (dronabinol) was the first synthetic THC approved for the treatment of nausea. Despite being approved by the FDA, and still available today, dronabinol does not appear to be nearly as effective as natural medical cannabis.

Medical Cannabis Used Today

Changes are finally beginning to happen even at the federal level. In April of 2018, the FDA approved the first cannabis-based treatment. Epidiolex is cannabidiol (CBD) derived from the *Cannabis sativa* plant, which is indicated for the use of seizures in children. With more states approving cannabis for medicinal use and more evidence of the benefits of cannabis being published, public opinion has started to shift as well. Former Speaker of the House John Boehner, who is about as far from being liberal as one can imagine, is now working on behalf of a lobbying firm that advocates for the legalization and medical use of marijuana. In states where medical cannabis is legal, an entire industry has developed where state-regulated growers, processors, and dispensaries provide patients with a wide variety of options to treat medical conditions.

Chapter 1 Notes

1. O'Shaughnessy, W. B. Extract from a Memoir on the Preparations of the Indian Hemp, or Gunjah, (Cannabis Indica) their effects on the Animal system in Health, and their utility in the Treatment of Tetanus and other Convulsive Diseases. *Journal of the Asiatic Society of Bengal* 1839: 8(94), 839.

2. Mechoulam, R., and Y. Gaony. A total synthesis of DL-Delta-1-Tetrahydrocannabinol, the active constituent of hashish. *J Am Chem Soc.* 1965 Jul 20: 87, 3273–5.

3. https://www.dea.gov/controlled-substances-act accessed 4/15/2020.

4. Downs D. The Science behind the DEA's Long War on Marijuana. *Scientific American* April 19, 2016. Accessed online https://www.scientificamerican.com/article/the-science-behind-the-dea-s-long-war-on-marijuana/4/15/2020.

Chapter 2:

The Endocannabinoid System

What Is the Endocannabinoid System (ECS)?

Our bodies are made up of a number of integrated systems that allow our bodies to function. You are likely familiar with the circulatory system (heart, blood, blood vessels), which has the primary function of delivering oxygen (via blood) to all the other tissues and organs in the body. There are many other systems such as the nervous system, respiratory system, endocrine system, et cetera. The endocannabinoid system (ECS) is a regulatory system in the body that has the primary function of assisting homeostasis. Homeostasis is a scientific term for keeping everything running smoothly and "status" quo. When things start going badly (stress, hunger, fatigue, and so forth) systems that help with homeostasis attempt to right the ship and keep things on track. There are multiple systems in our bodies that attempt to achieve homeostasis, so the ECS is not alone. However, research has found that the ECS has an important role in maintaining homeostasis in a variety of our body's important functions, including appetite, pain sensations, mood, immunity, and memory.[1]

The ECS is an evolutionary development that helped many species, including humans. Not only do all humans possess an endocannabinoid system, but all vertebrate species also have their own ECS. The endocannabinoid system has been around for about six hundred million years. Interestingly, the marijuana plant has only been around for twenty-five million years. In other words, vertebrate animals, including humans, did not evolve by creating the ECS to adapt to the properties of a plant. Rather, the story of the ECS and how medical cannabis works is much more about human and animal biology than about a plant that has been around a comparatively short time.

Like several other systems in our body, the ECS is comprised of messengers and receptors. Messengers are natural chemicals produced in the body (biochemicals) that hit certain receptors (often peptides, which are a series of amino acids) that, when combined, cause the flow of certain molecules across a cell membrane to produce an action. For example, beta receptors in the airways and in the heart respond to epinephrine (adrenaline), which is released during stress, which promote the lungs to take up more air and the heart to beat faster. In the case of the ECS, the messengers are called endocannabinoids, and the receptors are called cannabinoid receptors.

The Endocannabinoids

Endocannabinoids are chemical messengers that are mostly produced in the brain and can be classified as neurotransmitters. Neurotransmitters are the chemical messengers that relay messages from one nerve cell or neuron to another. There are many other neurotransmitters in our body that play a variety of roles. The main neurotransmitters in the brain are serotonin, dopamine, and norepinephrine. In patients with depression, levels of serotonin can be low, and doctors will sometimes use medications called serotonin reuptake inhibitors (SSRIs), which increase levels of serotonin in the nerve receptors. Nicotine increases brain levels of dopamine. One medication that has been used to help with smoking cessation is bupropion, which also increases dopamine in the brain. Thus, similar to other neurotransmitters in the body, the endocannabinoids can not only affect the body's function, but the use of molecules that are similar to the endocannabinoids or agents that interact to either increase or decrease endocannabinoids can also be useful in treating certain diseases.

There are two main endocannabinoids in the ECS: anandamide and 2-AG. They are synthesized primarily by the brain on an as-needed basis to help regulate processes in the body that maintain homeostasis. Anandamide plays a role in hunger/feeding, motivation, and pleasure. In one study, when anandamide was injected into the area of a rat's brain that deals with pleasure/rewards, it increased the rat's response to tasting sugar, as well as increasing food intake.[2] In fact, in certain disease states, such as fibromyalgia and migraine, researchers have found that individuals affected with these conditions have low levels of endocannabinoids compared to those without these medical conditions.[3] This concept of endocannabinoid deficiency is changing our understanding of several related diseases that many doctors and researchers continue to believe are mostly psychosomatic.

The Cannabinoid Receptors

For the ECS to work, endocannabinoids need to interact with cannabinoid receptors. There are two main cannabinoid receptors (CB) receptors found throughout the body: CB1 and CB2.[4] CB1 is located primarily in the brain and peripheral nervous system; CB2 can be found mainly in immune cells as well as other organs in the body, including the spleen, kidney, liver, and skin. CB2 receptors can also be found in the brain and nervous system, though to a much lesser extent. CB receptors are like many other receptors in the body. They are made of proteins and sit on the surface of a cell membrane. When stimulated by a messenger (in this case, anandamide or 2-AG), they open and/or close channels across the membrane that allow certain molecules to cross (for example, calcium), which in turn causes a response in that cell and therefore a response in the body. One of the interesting things about the CB receptors is that they are functionally selective.[4] This means that different messengers can have differing effects at the same receptor. This presents both opportunities and challenges when considering how to manipulate the ECS (either with plant products or synthetic medications) to improve health and treat disease.

Cannabis, CBD, and the ECS

In summary, the ECS is a naturally occurring system in our body that has been around for hundreds of millions of years, which helps regulate a variety of functions in our bodies to help keep things functioning normally (homeostasis). The ECS is comprised of two main endocannabinoids (anandamide and 2-AG), and two cannabinoid receptors (CB1 and CB2). So, what is the connection to marijuana (cannabis) and CBD (cannabidiol) and the ECS? As it turns out, there are other molecules that can interact with the CB receptors. These compounds are collectively known as cannabinoids. Anandamide and 2-AG are produced in the body and are thus called endocannabinoids, because they are endogenous (made in the body) cannabinoids. However, there are also exogenous cannabinoids. Marijuana, or cannabis, is a plant that contains many cannabinoids (CBD and THC being two of the main ones) that also interact with the CB receptors. Thus, marijuana as well as a related plant called hemp contain plant-based or phytocannabinoids. In addition, researchers have been able to synthesize cannabinoids that can affect the body as well. For example, dronabinol is a pharmaceutical agent that is a synthetic version of the phytocannabinoid THC. It has been available since the late '80s and has been used to treat severe nausea.

Using plant-based molecules to affect an endogenous system is not unique to the ECS. A similar system exists with opioids. Our body makes its own pain relievers, including endorphins and enkephalins, which are also neurotransmitters that react with our bodies' own natural opioid receptors in the brain to reduce pain. The poppy seed plant has been used to make opioids that can treat pain, and drug companies have been able to create synthetic opioids, such as oxycodone, which has been used to treat pain. Another similarity in this comparison is that the poppy seed plant can also be used to make opium or heroin, which is used as a recreational drug. Thus, even though marijuana can be used as a recreational drug, this doesn't mean it can't also be used, like the opioids, effectively as a medicine. Two very big differences between marijuana and narcotics are addiction and lethality. Narcotics are highly addictive and can be very lethal. Cannabis is minimally addictive (about the same as coffee), and essentially cannot lead to death.

Chapter 2 Notes

1. Aizpurua-Olaizola, O., I. Elezgarai, I. Rico-Barrio, I. Zarandona, N. Etxebarria, and A. Usobiaga. Targeting the endocannabinoid system: Future therapeutic strategies. *Drug Discovery Today* 2016, 22(1):105-110.

2. Pacher, P., S. Batkai, and G. Kunos. The Endocannabinoid System as an Emerging Target of Pharmacotherapy. *Pharmacol Rev* 2006: 58(3), 389–462.

3. Russo, Ethan B. "Clinical endocannabinoid deficiency reconsidered: current research supports the theory in migraine, fibromyalgia, irritable bowel, and other treatment-resistant syndromes." *Cannabis and cannabinoid research* 1.1. 2016: 154–165.

4. Mackie, K. Cannabinoid Receptors: Where They Are and What They Do. *Journal of Neuroendocrinology* 2008: 20(s1), 10–14.

Chapter 3:

Cannabinoids, Terpenes, and the Entourage Effect

Whole-Plant Medicine

Cannabis is a plant that has hundreds of ingredients that can affect your body in a number of different ways. This chapter will discuss cannabinoids and terpenes, as well as how they work together to produce unique medicinal effects on the body. One of the unique things about plant-based medicine, and cannabis and hemp in particular, is that using all of the components in the whole plant combined seems to work better than the individual components alone. As mentioned in the previous chapter, synthetic THC (dronabinol) has been around since the mideighties as a treatment for nausea. While it is still in limited use today, it is not viewed as very effective by many clinicians and patients. In contrast, the THC used with whole-plant cannabis seems to be much more effective, likely because of the other ingredients in the plant and how their combined interaction affects the body.

Cannabinoids

As mentioned in the previous chapter, cannabinoids are molecules that interact with cannabinoid receptors in the body to produce a variety of effects in the ECS to maintain homeostatic functions such as metabolism and sleep. The body produces two cannabinoids in the brain (anandamide and 2-AG), and because they are made internally in the body, they are referred to as endocannabinoids. However, there are a variety of cannabinoids that are not produced in the body that can also interact with cannabinoid receptors in the body. Pharmaceutical companies have made synthetic cannabinoids such as dronabinol, which have some medicinal effects. Fortunately, both cannabis and a version of cannabis called hemp contain naturally growing plant-based cannabinoids, which are also known as phytocannabinoids. While THC and CBD are the main phytocannabinoids associated with cannabis and hemp, both these plants contain a variety of other cannabinoids that have additional medicinal properties. In fact, there are over a hundred different cannabinoids that have been discovered in the cannabis plant with a variety of different properties.[1]

THC

THC is the abbreviated term for delta-9-tetrahydrocannabinol. THC was discovered by Dr. Raphael Mechoulam, an Israeli organic chemist at the Hebrew University of Jerusalem in 1964.[2] Dr. Mechoulam determined that THC was responsible the psychoactive effects of cannabis, as well as many of the medicinal properties. He also isolated the endocannabinoids anandamide and 2-AG and described the entire endocannabinoid system.

As stated in the previous section, THC affects the body by binding to and stimulating the CB1 and CB2 receptors in the body, mimicking the functions of the endocannabinoid anandamide. THC is responsible for the psychoactive effects in the brain, including causing euphoria, or the feeling of being "high," as well as other effects such as changes in mood, balance, coordination, memory, and appetite (see Table 1).

THC has been shown to have many therapeutic effects on the body and thus can work like a medicine for a variety of conditions such as relieving pain,[3] reducing inflammation,[4] helping with nausea, reducing symptoms of anxiety,[5] and treating seizure disorders[6] and glaucoma,[7] to name just a few. THC and other cannabinoids may also help protect the brain against injury, such as after a stroke or trauma.[8]

CBD

CBD stands for cannabidiol. Unlike THC, which directly interacts with the CB receptors, CBD has low affinity for the CB receptors. The effects of CBD are more related to decreasing the activity of other substans, including other cannabinoids, at the CB receptors.[9] When combined with THC, CBD can actually decrease the psychoactive and other properties of THC.[10] CBD is nonpsychoactive and does not cause sedation. This doesn't mean that CBD is the opposite of THC. Their effects can be both opposing and complementary (see Table 1). In addition, CBD has been shown to interact with other important receptors in the body that play a role in pain, anxiety, and depression, such as opioid receptors and serotonin receptors, and CBD has been shown to inhibit the reuptake of important neurotransmitters involved in these pathways, such as norepinephrine, dopamine, serotonin, and GABA.[11]

CBD is a popular cannabinoid used in both marijuana and hemp. Because of its popularity and increased use, an entire section of this book is devoted entirely to CBD. In summary, CBD is a nonpsychoactive cannabinoid that has medicinal properties both in conjunction with THC and other cannabinoids, as well as medicinal properties used on its own. CBD has been shown to be useful in a variety of conditions, including anxiety, depression, seizures, inflammation, and chronic pain.[12]

Table 1: Comparison of Medicinal Properties of THC and CBD

THC	CBD
Psychoactive	Nonpsychoactive
Sedation; induces sleep	Does not cause sedation
Primarily relieves pain; also decreases inflammation	Primarily decreases inflammation, also relieves pain

THC	CBD
Anxiety at high doses; relieves anxiety at low doses	Relieves anxiety and depression
Increases appetite	Suppresses appetite
Reduces seizures	Reduces seizures

CBG

All of the phytocannabinoids are derived from parent cannabinoid called cannabigerolic acid (CBGa). CBGa is the precursor to the acidic forms of THC and CBD, called THCa and CBDa, respectively. With heat and time, THCa and CBDa is converted to THC and CBD. Both the acid and nonacidic, or neutral, cannabinoids have effects on the body. CBG, or cannabigerol, is the nonacidic form of CBGa, and similarly gets converted with time and heat. In most cannabis plants, there is actually very little CBG, usually less than 1%. CBG is similar to CBD in that it also is nonpsychoactive. There is very little research into the effects of CBG on humans, though interest is growing, as it is thought that different nonpsychoactive cannabinoids may have many distinct clinical uses.

Animal studies have shown that CBG stimulates receptors involved in pain and heat sensation, can stimulate a2-adrenergic receptors in the brain and blood vessels, which are involved in blood pressure regulation, and can also block the uptake of neurotransmitters such as serotonin and norepinephrine.[13, 14] Thus, CBG might have a role in blood pressure regulation, anxiety/depression, and pain. Finally, CBG may have some anti-inflammatory properties as well.[15] All of these effects are also seen with CBD, so it is unclear whether or not CBG, which again is produced by the plant in much lower quantities, has any differentiating properties.

THCa

As mentioned, THCa is the nonpsychoactive acidic precursor to THC. Because heat will oxidize THCa into THC, THCa can only be used medicinally from nonheated cannabis. There is very little research on THCa. However it is reported to have anti-inflammatory properties,[16] as well as potential use in relieving nausea.[17]

CBDa

Like THCa, cannabidolic acid, or CBDa, is the acidic precursor to CBD and can only be obtained from nonheated cannabis plants. CBDa is found in the resin glands, or trichomes, of the raw cannabis plant. Like THCa, there is also limited research on CBDa. It is thought to have several properties, including being good for inflammation[18] and pain,[19] and being antibacterial.[20]

CBN

Over time, with or without heat, THC oxidizes and is converted into cannabinol (CBN). While CBN is less psychoactive than THC, it can be very sedating, and thus useful for sleep.[21] CBN may be useful for promoting sleep without causing any impairment. Because CBN is converted from THC, it is much easier to obtain. Therefore, it is more common in medical cannabis products that can be obtained in dispensaries, especially those specifically designed to help patients sleep.

CBC

CBC (Cannabichromene) is a lesser-known cannabinoid usually found in younger plants. While there is limited study on CBC, it has not been found to cause sedation.[22] Unlike CBD, CBC may actually enhance the effects of THC.[23] There are several reported medicinal benefits of CBC, including decreasing pain[24] and inflammation,[25] and having strong antimicrobial effects.[26]

Terpenes

In addition to the cannabinoids, cannabis and hemp plants also have substances called terpenes. Both cannabinoids and terpenes have effects on the body. Like the cannabinoids, the terpenes are produced from the glands, or trichomes, of the plant. Terpenes are plant-based oils that give many plants, including cannabis, their scent. Terpenes from other plants and fruits are the main components of essential oils that are also used therapeutically.[27] Over one hundred terpenes have been identified in the cannabis plant, with each strain having a unique terpene profile, usually with one or two terpenes being predominant in a particular strain.

While cannabinoids affect the body through interaction with the cannabinoid receptors (as well as other mechanism), terpenes affect the body through a variety of different mechanisms, which are just beginning to be discovered,[28] though we have known for some time that smell is an important sensation that connects to areas of the brain associated with emotion and memories. While there are many different terpenes in the plant kingdom, the most common terpenes found in cannabis and hemp are *alpha-pinene, beta-caryophyllene, humulene, limonene, linalool,* and *myrcene,* though there are many others (Table 2).

Alpha-Pinene

Alpha-Pinene is the most common terpene found in nature. It is found in pine trees and gives a pinelike scent to some strains of cannabis. It is also found in other plants such as rosemary and basil. It has been used as a bronchodilator to treat asthma, has antibacterial properties, and may help with memory.

Beta-Caryophyllene

Beta-caryophyllene is found in black pepper and has a peppery scent. It is also found in oregano, cloves, and green leafy vegetables. Beta-caryophyllene is cannabinoidlike because it has a strong affinity for the

CB2 receptors. Beta-caryophyllene is anti-inflammatory and may also help with nerve pain and protect the stomach.

Camphene

Camphene has a woodsy, musky, and pungent odor. It occurs naturally in many places, including rosemary, fir, lavender, sage, nutmeg, and ginger. It can be found in several essential oils such as turpentine, camphor oil, citronella oil, and ginger oil. Camphene is used as a flavoring for foods,in fragrances, and is used in topical creams to treat eczema and psoriasis. Interestingly, camphene may lower cholesterol.

Humulene

Humulene is found in hops as well as cannabis and is responsible for the aroma and taste of hoppy beers. The scent has been described as earthy, woody, spicy, and herbal. It has antitumor and anti-inflammatory properties and can also suppress appetite.

Limonene

Limonene is common in citrus fruits and thus gives off a citrus scent. It can also be found in peppermint and rosemary, as well as cannabis. Limonene has a variety of effects on the body, including fighting cancer, acting as an antidepressant or antianxiety agent, has antibacterial properties, and may help with heartburn (gastroesophageal reflux).

Linalool

Linalool is found in lavender and therefore has a lavenderlike scent. It can also be found in birch and other plants. It can cause sedation and thus is thought to be good for stress. Linalool also has analgesic and anticonvulsant properties.

Myrcene

Myrcene can be found in mangos, lemongrass, and hops, as well as cannabis. Its aroma has been described as earthy, fruity, and clovelike. The main properties of myrcene are sedation and muscle relaxation. It also has anti-inflammatory properties.

Ocimene

Ocimene can be found in mint, parsley, basil, and orchids and has a sweet aroma. Potential therapeutic benefits of ocimene include antiviral, antifungal, antiseptic, decongestant, and antibacterial properties; thus, it is a good terpene to use if you are sick.

Phellandrene

Phellandrene has a peppermintlike aroma and can be found in eucalyptus as well as a number of herbs and spices, including cinnamon, garlic, dill, ginger, and parsley. Phellandrene is also used as a food flavoring and in perfumes. It can be used to treat digestive disorders and has antifungal properties.

Pulegone

Pulegone is one of the lesser terpenes in cannabis. It has a peppermint aroma and can be found in rosemary. Pulegone has sedative and fever-reducing properties and may help with memory.

Sabinene

Sabinene has aromas of pine, orange, and spice. Sabinene occurs in many plants, including spruce, black pepper, and basil. Sabinene may have antioxidant and anti-inflammatory properties.

Terpinolene

Terpinolene has a floral aroma and can be found in apples, lilacs, and nutmeg; it is commonly used in soaps and perfumes and is known to be sedating. It also has antioxidant, antibacterial, antifungal, and anticancer properties.

Table 2: Terpenes and Their Properties

Terpene	Aroma	Therapeutic Effect
Alpha-Pinene	Pine	Bronchodilator, antibacterial, memory
Beta-caryophyllene	Pepper	Anti-inflammatory, nerve pain
Camphene	Woodsy/musky	Anti-inflammatory, may lower cholesterol
Humulene	Hoppy	Antitumor, anti-inflammatory, appetite suppressant
Limonene	Citrus	Antitumor, antidepressant/ anxiety, antibacterial properties, heartburn
Linalool	Lavender	Sedative, analgesic, anticonvulsant, stress
Myrcene	Clove/fruity	Sedative, muscle relaxant, anti-inflammatory

Terpene	Aroma	Therapeutic Effect
Ocimene	Sweet	Antiviral, antifungal, antiseptic, decongestant, and antibacterial
Phellandrene	Peppermint	Antifungal, digestive disorders
Pulegone	Peppermint	Sedative, fever reducing, memory
Sabinene	Pine/orange/spice	Antioxidant, anti-inflammatory
Terpinolene	Floral	Sedative, antioxidant, antibacterial, antifungal, antitumor

The Entourage Effect

With so many cannabinoids and terpenes, the mechanisms of cannabis on the body may seem rather complicated. However, the mechanism of action of cannabis on the body is even more complex than just cannabinoids and terpenes. We have reviewed the cannabinoids, which interact with CB receptors in the body and how they affect the ECS. We have discussed terpenes, which are the aromatic compounds in cannabis that can affect the body in a variety of ways. There are also other components in cannabis that have effects on the body. For example, flavonoids are compounds that give pigment and color to plants like cannabis as well as flowers, and they may also have unique medicinal properties. However, one interesting fact about cannabis is that the sum of all of these components (cannabinoids, terpenes, flavonoids, et cetera) appears to be greater the effects of their individual properties combined. It is not just the various cannabinoids and terpenes in the cannabis plant that affect the body, but it is how they work in combination to achieve their healing properties.

For most medications, a drug is designed to interact with a particular receptor to produce a desired effect. For example, opioids like oxycodone interact with our own natural opioid receptors in the brain to produce pain relief. While it is true that cannabinoids such as THC interact with CB receptors to also produce pain relief, the other components of cannabis (other cannabinoids, terpenes, et cetera) significantly modulate this effect. For example, CBD can decrease some of the psychoactive properties of THC when administered together. As mentioned, synthetic THC (dronabinol) was developed in 1985 for nausea. While there is no randomized trial that compares cannabis and dronabinol, dronabinol is not felt to be nearly as effective as cannabis for the use of nausea.

In one study, scientists compared the antitumor properties of pure THC compared to a whole-plant extract in both animals and cell cultures on the effect of breast cancer cells. They found that the whole-plant extract was far more potent than the THC alone.[29] Also, as we will discuss in the chapter on CBD, while increasing the dose of isolated CBD increases the effectiveness, it also increases the number of side effects. This doesn't happen when using the entire CBD-rich hemp plant extract.[30] This ability of all the components of the cannabis and hemp plant to work together, and synergistically affect the body in ways that are both complementary and exceed the benefits of each of the individual components in the plant, is known as the "entourage effect."[27] In other words, it is not just the celebrity THC that is important, but its entire "entourage" of additional cannabinoids, terpenes, and flavonoids that are needed to produce the overall results. In the section regarding using medical cannabis, we will discuss how various different strains of the cannabis plant are used to treat specific medical conditions. For example, some cannabis strains are best for anxiety, while other strains are best for pain relief. While the amounts of THC and CBD are important, it is the entourage effect of the various different cannabis strains that explain their different medicinal properties. This variation of components and the entourage effect allows clinicians and patients to select the most appropriate strains of the cannabis plant to treat a particular ailment.

Chapter 3 Notes

1. Aizpurua-Olaizola, O., U. Soydaner, E. Öztürk, et al. Evolution of the Cannabinoid and Terpene Content during the Growth of Cannabis sativa Plants from Different Chemotypes. *Journal of Natural Products* 2016: 79(2), 324–331.

2. Gaoni, Y., and R. Mechoulam. Isolation, Structure, and Partial Synthesis of an Active Constituent of Hashish. *J. Am. Chem. Soc.* 1964: 86(8), 1646–1647.

3. Noyes, R., et al. "The analgesic properties of delta-9-tetrahydrocannabinol." *Clin Pharmacol Ther* 1975: 18(1), 84–89.

4. Hammell, D., L. Zhang, F. Ma, F., et al. Transdermal cannabidiol reduces inflammation and pain-related behaviours in a rat model of arthritis. *European Journal of Pain* 2015: 20(6), 936–948.

5. Schier, A., N. Ribeiro, et al. Antidepressant-Like and Anxiolytic-Like Effects of Cannabidiol: A Chemical Compound of Cannabis sativa. *CNS & Neurological Disorders–Drug Targets* 2014: 13(6), 953–960.

6. Devinsky, O., J. Cross, L. Laux, E. Marsh, et al. Trial of Cannabidiol for Drug-Resistant Seizures in the Dravet Syndrome. *New England Journal of Medicine* 2017: 376(21), 2011–2020.

7. Adelli, G., P. Bhagav, P. Taskar, et al. Development of a Δ9-Tetrahydrocannabinol Amino Acid-Dicarboxylate Prodrug With Improved Ocular Bioavailability. *Invest Ophthalmol Vis Sci.* 2017 Apr: 58(4), 2167–2179.

8. Mechoulam, R., D. Panikashvili, and E. Shohami. "Cannabinoids and brain injury: therapeutic implications." *Trends in molecular medicine* 2002: 8(2), 58–61.

9. Russo, E., A. Mead, and D. Sulak. Current and Future Status of Cannabis Research. *Clinical Researcher* 2015: 29(2), 58–63.

10. Russo, E., and W. G. Geoffrey. A tale of two cannabinoids: the therapeutic rationale for combining tetrahydrocannabinol and cannabidiol. *Medical hypotheses* 2006: 66(2), 234–246.

11. Zhornitsky, S., and S. Potvin. Cannabidiol in humans—the quest for therapeutic targets. *Pharmaceuticals* 2012: 5(5), 529–552.

12. Zuardi, A. W. Cannabidiol: from an inactive cannabinoid to a drug with wide spectrum of action. *Revista brasileira de psiquiatria* 2008: 30(3), 271–280.

13. Cascio, M. G., et al. Evidence that the plant cannabinoid cannabigerol is a highly potent α2-adrenoceptor agonist and moderately potent 5HT1A receptor antagonist. *British journal of pharmacology* 2010: (159)1, 129–141.

14. Banerjee, S. P., S. H. Snyder, and R. Mechoulam. Cannabinoids: influence on neurotransmitter uptake in rat brain synaptosomes. *J Pharmacol Exper Therap* 1975: (194), 74–81.

15. Evans, F. J. Cannabinoids: the separation of central from peripheral effects on a structural basis. *Planta Med* 1991: 57(Suppl 1), S60–7.

16. Ruhaak, L., J. Felth, P. Karlsson, J. Rafter, R. Verpoorte, and L. Bohlin. Evaluation of the Cyclooxygenase Inhibiting Effects of Six Major Cannabinoids Isolated from Cannabis sativa. *Biological & Pharmaceutical Bulletin* 2011: 34(5),]774–778.

17. Rock, E. M., et al. Tetrahydrocannabinolic acid reduces nausea-induced conditioned gaping in rats and vomiting in Suncus murinus. *British journal of pharmacology* 2013: 170(3), 641–648.

18. Takeda, S., et al. Cannabidiolic acid as a selective cyclooxygenase-2 inhibitory component in cannabis. *Drug metabolism and disposition* 2008: 36(9), 1917–1921.

19. Ampson, A., M. Grimaldi, M. Lolic, D. Wink, R. Rosenthal, and J. Axelrod. Neuroprotective Antioxidants from Marijuana. *Annals of the New York Academy of Sciences* 2006: 899(1), 274–282.

20. Izzo, A., F. Borrelli, R. Capasso, V. Di Marzo, and R. Mechoulam. Non-psychotropic plant cannabinoids: new therapeutic opportunities from an ancient herb. *Trends in Pharmacological Sciences* [online] 2009: 30(10), 515–527.

21. Huestis, M. A. Pharmacokinetics and Metabolism of the Plant Cannabinoids, Δ 9-Tetrahydrocannibinol, Cannabidiol and Cannabinol. *Cannabinoids.* Springer Berlin Heidelberg 2005, 657–690.

22. Turner, C. E., M. A. Elsohly, and E. G. Boeren. Constituents of Cannabis sativa L. XVII. A review of the natural constituents. *J Nat Prod* 1980: 43, 169–304.

23. O'Neil, J. D., W. S. Dalton, and R. B. Forney. The effect of cannabichromene on mean blood pressure, heart rate, and respiration rate responses to tetrahydrocannabinol in the anesthetized rat. *Toxicol Appl Pharmacol* 1979: 49, 265–70.

24. Davis, W. M., and N. S. Hatoum. Neurobehavioral actions of cannabichromene and interactions with Æ9-tetrahydrocannabinol. *Gen Pharmacol* 1993: 14(2), 247–52.

25. Wirth, P. W., E. S. Watson, M. ElSohly, C. E. Turner, and J. C. Murphy. Anti-inflammatory properties of cannabichromene. *Life Sci* 1980: 26, 1991–5.

26. ElSohly, H. N., C. E. Turner, A. M. Clark, and M. A. ElSohly. Synthesis and antimicrobial activities of certain cannabichromene and cannabigerol related compounds. *J Pharmaceut Sci* 1982: 71, 1319–23.

27. Russo, E. B. Taming THC: potential cannabis synergy and phytocannabinoid-terpenoid entourage effects. *Br J Pharmacol* 2011: 163(7), 1344–64.

28. Fischedick, J. E. Cannabinoids and Terpenes as Chemotaxonomic Markers in Cannabis. *Nat Prod Chem Res* 2015: 3(4), 1–9.

29. Blasco-Benitoab, S., M. Seijo-Vilaab, M. Caro-Villalobosa, et al. Appraising the "entourage effect": Antitumor action of a pure cannabinoid versus a botanical drug preparation in preclinical models of breast cancer. *Biochemical Pharmacology* 2018: 157, 285–293.

30. Gallily, R., Y. Zhannah, et al. Overcoming the Bell-Shaped Dose-Response of Cannabidiol by Using Cannabis Extract Enriched in Cannabidiol. *Pharmacology & Pharmacy* 2015: 6, 75–78.

Chapter 4:

The Science of Medical Cannabis

Medical Cannabis Research

In the previous section, we discussed the endocannabinoid system and the effect of cannabinoids, both endogenous and exogenous (i.e., the phytocannabinoids or medical cannabis), which is all based on a tremendous amount of research from all over the world. However, while there certainly is a vast amount of science behind the way in which cannabis works, there is also research regarding how cannabis can help treat disease. As mentioned, the federal status of marijuana has greatly limited the amount of research into this important therapeutic agent. The NIH spends hundreds of millions of dollars researching important diseases like cancer and infectious diseases, and the biopharmaceutical industry spends even more on research that brings therapeutic agents (drugs, vaccines, devices) to market in order to help patients. Since marijuana is federally illegal, those normal research institutions and industries simply cannot do the kind of research necessary to determine how to best use medical cannabis for patients. That said, through independent research and other sources around the world, there is enough research, both in animals and in humans, that confirms that medical cannabis is beneficial in a variety of different diseases.

Medical Cannabis: The Evidence to Date

In many areas of medicine, experts in a particular field of medicine from leading organizations (think cardiologists from the American Heart Association) will gather from across the country and review all of the available research to make recommendations or guidelines. When you hear reports in the media about new guidelines for high blood pressure or new recommendations for colon cancer screening, these reports are based on these types of scientific reviews. Fortunately, such a scientific review was done for medical cannabis. The National Academies of Sciences, Engineering, and Medicine performed such an analysis, titled "Health Effects of Cannabis and Cannabinoids: Current State of Evidence and Recommendations for Research."[1] The committee was made up of researchers from academic institutions from across the country and was sponsored by multiple public and private organizations, including the CDC, FDA, and the Robert W. Woodruff Foundation. They scoured multiple sources to find all the relevant research they could, looking at over twenty-four thousand publications. They focused their efforts on what they considered the highest-quality evidence and focused on eleven important areas of health, including cancer, heart disease, and mental health. From this research, in regard to treating diseases with medical cannabis, they concluded that there was valid, scientific evidence that clearly supported the use of medical cannabis in three areas:

1. In adults with chemotherapy-induced nausea and vomiting, oral cannabinoids are effective antiemetics (antinausea agents).
2. In adults with chronic pain, patients who were treated with cannabis or cannabinoids are more likely to experience a clinically significant reduction in pain symptoms.
3. In adults with multiple sclerosis (MS)–related spasticity, short-term use of oral cannabinoids improves patient-reported spasticity symptoms.

They also stated that for these conditions, the effects of cannabinoids were modest, and that for all other conditions evaluated, there is inadequate information to assess their effects. Now, this does not mean that cannabis doesn't work for other conditions. Rather, when looking at the highest quality of evidence typically used to make medical decisions, there was support for the use of medical cannabis in at least these three areas, but not enough high-quality evidence to make recommendations in support of other diseases. Given this high standard and the fact that research is so limited due to federal regulations, this report should give practitioners solid scientific ground for recommending medical cannabis and should be enough evidence for even skeptical clinicians to at least consider medical cannabis as an alternative treatment for certain conditions. This is especially important in the treatment of pain, given the large number of patients in this country who are using narcotics to treat chronic pain. The following sections review some of the research for these conditions, as well as some other conditions for which cannabis is commonly used to treat medical conditions. Please note that this chapter is not intended to be an extensive review of all the scientific research to date for medical cannabis, as the focus of this book is for patients to understand how to use medical cannabis for their conditions. In addition, there are several existing books that review the science of medical cannabis.

Medical Cannabis for Nausea

One of the first areas that the Academy of Sciences report supported was use of medical marijuana for nausea, specifically regarding nausea that is a side effect of cancer patients taking chemotherapy. Nausea is unfortunately a very common side effect of many chemotherapies used to treat many types of cancers. There are a variety of prescription medications commonly used for nausea, like Zofran (generic name is ondansetron), which can be very effective but may not always work for nausea induced by cancer.[2] Marinol (dronabinol) is a synthetic form of THC and was approved in the United States in 1985 for use in patients with chemotherapy-induced nausea. However, while it was somewhat effective, an analysis of multiple trials of Marinol and other synthetic cannabinoids found that they weren't much better than conventional medications.[3] However, there are several studies using cannabis extracts that have been shown to be effective for chemotherapy-induced nausea, and possibly more effective than the synthetic versions.[4] This is of interest, as it demonstrates that extracts of the plant itself seem to be more beneficial than synthetic derivatives, supporting the value of whole-plant-based medicine and the entourage effect. Clearly, more research is warranted into finding the best strains and formulations for use of medical cannabis in these patients.

Medical Cannabis for Pain

Pain is complex. There are different types of pain from different causes. Pain involves the brain, the spinal cord, and nerves that go from the spinal cord to the rest of the body called peripheral nerves. We also have two types of nervous systems in our body: the sympathetic nervous system, which helps us jump to action when we are in danger, and the parasympathetic nervous system, which helps run some of the resting functions of the body, like digestion. Stimulation of the cannabinoid receptors (CB1) can affect the sympathetic nervous system by blocking the release of norepinephrine (also known as adrenaline), dampen sympathetically mediated pain, and modulate some of the hormones, like cortisol, that can affect pain. There are also similarities in how opioids and cannabinoids work to treat pain. Just as the body makes endocannabinoids, the body also makes its own natural opioids called enkephalins. CB receptors and opioid receptors are also found in similar parts of the nervous system. In fact, studies have shown that blocking the breakdown of these natural pain relievers can be effective in treating pain.[5]

While pain is complex, the data on medical cannabis for pain, particularly chronic pain, is much clearer. In one study, looking at prescription data for Medicare enrollees (Medicare Part D), there was a reduction in the number of pain prescriptions in states where medical cannabis was legalized, with doctors writing 1,826 fewer pain prescriptions on average per year in states where medical cannabis was legal compared to doctors in nonlegal states.[6] In another study looking at deaths from opioid overdoses, from 1999–2010, it showed that in states where medical cannabis was legal, there was a 24.8% lower rate of death from opiate overdoses than states where medical cannabis was not legalized.[7]

While these studies reveal that the legalization of medical cannabis correlates to fewer pain prescriptions written and fewer deaths for opioid overdose, the real evidence that medical cannabis can help with pain in individuals comes from clinical trials. Clinical trials are studies in which patients with a disease are randomized to the agent in question (in this case, medical cannabis) and a placebo, or sugar pill, to ensure the agent actually works.

One analysis of multiple clinical trials[8] using medical cannabis for pain, reviewed twenty-eight randomized trials in patients with chronic pain (2,454 participants), most of which looked at plant-derived cannabinoids (standardized herbal preparations or flower), and all but one that compared patients to placebo. Most of these chronic pain trials were related to neuropathy (seventeen trials), but included other conditions such as cancer pain, multiple sclerosis, and rheumatoid arthritis. Though the trials were small and had some important differences, data analyzed from seven trials found that medical cannabis increased the likelihood that patients would experience pain relief by 40%, and data from six trials showed a greater reduction in numerical pain scores. There were also several smaller trials that show that patients who take narcotics (opioids) for chronic pain can actually lower their opioid dose if they use medical cannabis.[9, 10] Medical cannabis has also been shown to be effective in at least one study in reducing pain after surgery.[11]

Medical Cannabis in Mental Health Disorders

While the review done by the National Academies of Sciences, Engineering, and Medicine did not agree that there was sufficient high-quality evidence of benefit from medical cannabis in mental health disorders, in addition to chronic pain, mental health—anxiety in particular—is one of the most common conditions for which I treat patients using medical cannabis. While I have plenty of anecdotal evidence that medical cannabis can be quite effective in a variety of mental health conditions, there is certainly scientific evidence to back this up.

THC at high doses can induce anxiety and psychotic symptoms in healthy individuals.[12] In fact, some patients I have treated with medical cannabis have told me they were reluctant to use it because when they tried marijuana as a young adult for recreational purposes, it made them anxious or paranoid. This is likely because the dose of THC they got from "smoking pot" was too high. While high doses of THC can cause anxiety (anxiogenic), lower doses of THC can reduce anxiety (anxiolytic).

There are only limited clinical studies on the effects of cannabis on treating mood disorders. THC, when given to patients suffering from cancer, has been shown to have anxiolytic as well as antidepressant effects.[13] For patients with generalized anxiety disorder, nabilone, a synthetic version of THC not available in the United States, was more effective than placebo in reducing anxiety symptoms.[14] Post-traumatic stress disorder (PTSD) is related to anxiety, and in one study of eighty patients with PTSD, researchers found a 75% reduction in PTSD-related symptoms when using cannabis.[15]

CBD, which is the nonpsychoactive component of medical cannabis and also found in hemp-based formulations, also has anxiolytic properties. CBD may help with anxiety by decreasing the uptake of certain neurotransmitters in the brain, similar to the way prescription medications work. In addition, one small study showed that CBD-induced reductions in anxiety was related to changes in blood flow in different parts of the brain.[16] While there are a few small studies that show high-dose CBD might reduce acute anxiety before a stressful event, such as public speaking,[17] CBD has better evidence if taken on a daily basis, at lower doses (around 25 mg daily), to reduce general anxiety.[18] PTSD is related to anxiety, and in one small study, there was significant improvement in symptoms when patients with PTSD took daily CBD.[19]

Medical cannabis and CBD can also be useful for other mental health conditions such as depression. In regard to depression, the evidence for medical cannabis is both limited and shows mixed results.[20] There is slightly more evidence to support the use of CBD in depression. However, research on both animals and humans indicate that CBD may have antidepressant properties as well.[21, 22] Other areas where there are limited but mixed results include bipolar disorder, obsessive compulsive disease, and Tourette's syndrome.[20]

The effects of any psychoactive agent, including prescription medications, on the brain can be complex. Thus, when treating mental health disorders with medical cannabis, even at low doses, one must proceed with caution. As mentioned, in high enough doses, THC can increase anxiety. Research has indicated that there is at least a statistical association between cannabis use and the development of schizophrenia or other psychoses, with the highest risk among the most frequent users. In addition, at least in the recreational literature, heavy marijuana use can increase the risk for developing social anxiety disorders and suicidal ideation. However, since medicinal doses of medical cannabis are generally much lower than recreational doses, it's unclear whether these risks are applicable. Nonetheless, caution is always warranted.

Medical Cannabis and Cancer

Cancer may be the single most important disease where medical cannabis can help afflicted patients. Not only is there robust research for treating chemotherapy-induced nausea, but there is also promising early research for treating and even preventing cancer. There are essentially four ways to think about medical marijuana in patients with cancer: treating the symptoms of cancer, treating the side effects from cancer treatment, treating the cancer itself, and preventing cancer.

When cancer spreads throughout the body, it can cause a variety of symptoms, including pain in the places it has spread to, weight loss and wasting, and even anxiety related to having cancer. In a study of 177 cancer patients with pain not well controlled by even opioids, a cannabis extract significantly reduced pain scores compared to a placebo.[23] Similar findings were seen in a pharmaceutical-grade formulation of cannabinoids not available in the United States,[24] and a group of doctors in Nevada found that in a group of 25 patients treated with long-term opioids for cancer-related pain, they were able to reduce opioid dose by at least half in almost all of these patients.[25] Cannabis has also been shown to have some potential value in treating cancer patients with loss of appetite and weight loss,[26, 27] as well as anxiety.[13]

Sometimes the side effects of cancer treatment, chemotherapy in particular, can be worse than the cancer itself. As mentioned, the National Academies of Sciences, Engineering, and Medicine found robust data in their review to support the use of medical cannabis to reduce nausea associated with chemotherapy.[1] Neuropathy, which is pain and/or tingling usually in the extremities, is another side effect of chemotherapy, which can persist after treatment and in some cases may become permanent. Because of the concentration of CB1 receptors on nerve cells, medical cannabis can be effective in treating and even preventing postchemotherapy neuropathy. While clinical studies demonstrating the benefit of treating neuropathy in human patients are not yet published as of this writing, in animal studies, when given CBD in advance of and during the administration of the chemotherapeutic agent paclitaxel, there was a reduction in neuropathic pain.[28]

Perhaps the greatest potential for use of cannabis in patients with cancer is treating the cancer itself. Cannabis has been shown in laboratory studies to turn on switches that cause cancer cells to die, prevent cancer cells from metastasizing, limit the growth of cancer cells, and prevent a process called angiogenesis, which is where cancer cells make their own blood vessels to help them get nourishment and grow.[29, 30, 31] Even more importantly, the anticancer effects of cannabinoids appear to treat cancer without harming healthy surrounding tissue.[32] There is even laboratory evidence that combining cannabis with traditional chemotherapy enhances the effects of the chemotherapy, potentially allowing for lower doses of chemotherapy and therefore fewer side effects.[33] Unfortunately, given the federal laws that limit the ability to do research, large trials of cannabis as a cancer treatment in humans are not yet available. However, there are some anecdotal reports of high-dose cannabis treatments being effective for certain patients with cancer.[34, 35]

Finally, in addition to treating cancer with cannabis, because of its anticancer effects, cannabis may be effective in preventing cancer from occurring in the first place. Mice can be bred to be predisposed to developing certain kinds of cancer. In two studies, one for colon cancer[36] and another for lung cancer,[37] mice that were bred to be genetically predisposed to theses cancers were much less likely to develop those cancers than similar mice that did not receive cannabis. While this may not be applicable to humans, in at least one study of over eighty thousand men showed that men who used cannabis but not tobacco had a 45% reduced risk of bladder cancer.[38]

Medical Cannabis in the Elderly

Medical cannabis and CBD appear to have great benefit for chronic pain, anxiety, and sleep, all very common issues in the elderly. In addition, as we age, we are affected with more and more medical conditions, which usually require more and more medications. Since prescription medications generally have interactions, using multiple medications (polypharmacy) in the elderly can sometime lead to problems. The benefit of a plant-based medicine is that it can often treat a variety of conditions at once, thus limiting the need for multiple medications and reducing issues with polypharmacy. Thus, the uses of medical cannabis and CBD in the elderly may have particular value.

While there is extremely limited research using medical cannabis in the elderly, there is one important study worth mentioning.[39] This study is important due to its large size (2,736 participants) and that the study was done in patients sixty-five years of age and older, which is not usually an easy population to enroll in clinical trials. In addition, the focus on the study was not only how well cannabis worked (efficacy), but also looked at safety issues. This was a prospective study in seniors receiving medical cannabis from January 2015 through October 2017, for a variety of conditions, the most common being cancer-related pain. Almost all patients (97%) reported improvements in their condition. For patients with pain, pain was reduced from an average rating of 8 (on a zero to 10 scale, with 10 being the worst), to 4. After six months, 18% of patients were able to stop or reduce their opioid dose. Perhaps more important than the benefits of medical cannabis in the elderly seen in this study was the low number of side effects. The most common side effects were dizziness (9.7%), dry mouth (7.1%), somnolence (3.9%), weakness (2.3%), and nausea (2.2%). All other effects were pretty rare (less than 2%). Other than dizziness and dry mouth, side effects of cannabis in this large population of elderly patients were fairly low, and comparable to or better than the side effects of many common prescription medications. While dizziness is certainly a concern, as falls in the elderly can be serious, an observational study of 204 patients of seventy-five years of age and older enrolled in New York State's Medical Marijuana Program showed no increased risk of falls.[40] Given the potential benefit of helping with several common ailments of elderly patients, the ability of whole-plant medicines to reduce the number of prescriptions needed, the low risk of adverse reactions seen in a relatively large study, and limited interactions with other medications, the use of medical cannabis in the elderly has a huge potential for benefit in this patient population.

Chapter 4 Notes

1. National Academies of Sciences, Engineering, and Medicine. 2017. The Health Effects of Cannabis and Cannabinoids: The Current State of Evidence and Recommendations for Research. Washington, DC: The National Academies Press. https://doi.org/10.17226/24625.

2. Ranganath, R., L. Einhorn, and C. Albany. Management of Chemotherapy Induced Nausea and Vomiting in Patients on Multiday Cisplatin Based Combination Chemotherapy. *Biomed Res Int*. 2015: 943618.

3. Smith, L. A., F. Azariah, T. C. V. Lavender, N. S. Stoner, and S. Bettiol. Cannabinoids for nausea and vomiting in adults with cancer receiving chemotherapy. *Cochrane Database of Systematic Reviews* 2015: (11), CD009464.

4. Mortimer, T. L., T. Mabin, and A. Engelbrecht. Cannabinoids: the lows and the highs of chemotherapy-induced nausea and vomiting. *Future Oncology* 2019: 15(9), 1035–1049.

5. Roques, B. P., M. C. Fournié-Zaluski, and M. Wurm. Inhibiting the breakdown of endogenous opioids and cannabinoids to alleviate pain. *Nat Rev Drug Discov* 2012 Apr: 11(4), 292–310.

6. Bradford, A. C., and W. D. Bradford. Medical marijuana laws reduce prescription medication use in Medicare part D. *Health Affairs* 2016: 35(7),1230–1236.

7. Bachhuber, M. A., B. Saloner, C. O. Cunningham, et al. Medical Cannabis Laws and Opioid Analgesic Overdose Mortality in the United States, 1999–2010. *JAMA Intern Med*. 2014: 174(10), 1668–1673.

8. Whiting, P. F., R. F. Wolff, S. Deshpande, et al. Cannabinoids for Medical Use. A Systematic Review and Meta-analysis. *JAMA* 2015 Jun 23–30: 313(24), 2456–73.

9. Boehnke, K. F., E. Litinas, and D. J. Clauw. Medical Cannabis Use Is Associated With Decreased Opiate Medication Use in a Retrospective Cross-Sectional Survey of Patients With Chronic Pain. *J Pain*. 2016 Jun: 17(6), 739–44.

10. Abrams, D. I., P. Couey, S. B. Shade, et al. Cannabinoid-opioid interaction in chronic pain. *Clin Pharmacol Ther.* 2011 Dec: 90(6), 844–51.

11. Holdcroft, A., M. Maze, C. Doré, S. Tebbs, and S. A. Thompson. A multicenter dose-escalation study of the analgesic and adverse effects of an oral cannabis extract (Cannador) for postoperative pain management. *Anesthesiology* 01 May 2006: 104(5), 1040–1046.

12. D'Souza, D. C., E. Perry, L. MacDougall, et al. The psychotomimetic effects of intravenous delta-9-tetrahydrocannabinol in healthy individuals: Implications for psychosis. *Neuropsychopharmacology* 2004: 29(8), 1558–1572.

13. Regelson, W., J. R. Butler, J. Schulz, T. Kirk, L. Peek, M. L. Green, and M. O. Zalis. Delta 9-THC as an effective antidepressant and appetite-stimulating agent in advanced cancer patients. In M. C. Braude and S. Szara (Eds.), *The Pharmacology of Marihuana* 1976, 763–776. New York: Raven Press.

14. Fabre, L. F., and D. McLendon. The efficacy and safety of nabilone (a synthetic cannabinoid) in the treatment of anxiety. *J Clin Pharmacol.* 1981 Aug–Sep: 21(S1), 377S–382S.

15. Greer, G. R., Grob, C. S., and A. L. Halberstadt. PTSD symptom reports of patients evaluated for the New Mexico Medical Cannabis Program. *J Psychoactive Drugs* 2014 Jan–Mar: 46(1), 73–7.

16. Crippa, J. A., G. N. Derenusson, T. B. Ferrari, et al. Neural basis of anxiolytic effects of cannabidiol (CBD) in generalized social anxiety disorder: a preliminary report. *J Psychopharmacol* 2011 Jan: 25(1),121–30.

17. Bergamaschi, M. M., R. H. Queiroz, et al. Cannabidiol reduces the anxiety induced by simulated public speaking in treatment-naïve social phobia patients. *Neuropsychopharmacology* 2011 May: 36(6), 1219–26.

18. Shannon, S., et al. Cannabidiol in Anxiety and Sleep: A Large Case Series. *Perm J* 2019: 23, 18–41.

19. Elms, L., S. Shannon, S. Hughes, and N. Lewis. Cannabidiol in the Treatment of Post-Traumatic Stress Disorder: A Case Series. *Journal of Alternative & Complementary Medicine* 2019 Apr: 25(4), 392–397.

20. Turna, J., B. Patterson, and M. Van Ameringen. Is cannabis treatment for anxiety, mood, and related disorders ready for prime time? *Depression and Anxiety* 2017: 34(11), 1006–1017.

21. Hill, M. N., and B. B. Gorzalka. The endocannabinoid system and the treatment of mood and anxiety disorders. *CNS Neurol Disord Drug Targets* 2009 Dec: 8(6), 451–8.

22. de Mello Schier, A.R., N. P. de Oliveira Ribeiro, et al. Antidepressant-like and anxiolytic-like effects of cannabidiol: a chemical compound of Cannabis sativa. *CNS Neurol Disord Drug Targets* 2014: 13(6), 953–60.

23. Johnson, J. R., M. Burnell-Nugent, D. Lossignol, et al. Multicenter, double-blind, randomized, placebo-controlled, parallel-group study of the efficacy, safety, and tolerability of THC: CBD extract and THC extract in patients with intractable cancer-related pain. *J Pain Symptom Manage* 2010 Feb: 39(2), 167–79.

24. Portenoy, R. K., et al. Nabiximols for opioid-treated cancer patients with poorly-controlled chronic pain: a randomized, placebo-controlled, graded-dose trial. *The Journal of Pain* 2012: 13(5), 438–449.

25. Teoh, D., T. J. Smith, M. Song, N. M. Spirtos. Care After Chemotherapy: Peripheral Neuropathy, Cannabis for Symptom Control, and Mindfulness. *Am Soc Clin Oncol Educ Book* 2018 May: 23(38), 469–479.

26. Abrams, D. I., and M. Guzman. Cannabis in cancer care. *Clinical Pharmacology & Therapeutics* 2015: 97(6), 575–586.

27. Jatoi, A., H. E. Windschitl, C. L. Loprinzi, et al. Dronabinol versus megestrol acetate versus combination therapy for cancer-associated anorexia: a North Central Cancer Treatment Group study. *J Clin Oncol.* 2002 Jan 15: 20(2), 567–73.

28. Ward, S. J., S. D. McAllister, H. Neelakantan, and E. A. Walker. Cannabidiol inhibits paclitaxel-induced neuropathic pain through 5-HT1A receptors without diminishing nervous system function or chemotherapy efficacy. *Br. J. Pharmacol.* 2014: 171, 636–645.

29. Munson, A. E., L. S. Harris, M. A. Friedman, W. L. Dewey, and R. A. Carchman. Antineoplastic Activity of Cannabinoids. *JNCI: Journal of the National Cancer Institute* 1975 Sep: 55(3), 597–602.

30. National Toxicology Program. NTP Toxicology and Carcinogenesis Studies of 1-Trans-Delta(9)-Tetrahydrocannabinol (CAS No. 1972-08-3) in F344 Rats and B6C3F1 Mice (Gavage Studies). *Natl Toxicol Program Tech Rep Ser.* 1996 Nov: 446, 1–317

31. Ladin, D. A., et al. Preclinical and clinical assessment of cannabinoids as anti-cancer agents. *Frontiers in pharmacology* 2016: 7, 361.

32. Galve-Roperh, I., C. Sánchez, M. L. Cortés, T. Gómez del Pulgar, M. Izquierdo, and M. Guzmán. Anti-tumoral action of cannabinoids: involvement of sustained ceramide accumulation and extracellular signal-regulated kinase activation. *Nat Med.* 2000 Mar: 6(3), 313–9.

33. Scott, K. A., A. G. Dalgleish, and W. M. Liu. Anticancer effects of phytocannabinoids used with chemotherapy in leukaemia cells can be improved by altering the sequence of their administration. *International Journal of Oncology* 2017: 51(1), 369–377.

34. Singh, Y., and B. Chamandeep. Cannabis Extract Treatment for Terminal Acute Lymphoblastic Leukemia with a Philadelphia Chromosome Mutation. *Case reports in oncology* 2013: 6(3), 585–592.

35. Kander, J. *Cannabis for the Treatment of Cancer: The Anticancer Activity of Phytocannabinoids and Endocannabinoids*, 4th edition, 2017.

36. Aviello, G., B. Romano, F. Borrelli, et al. Chemopreventive effect of the non-psychotropic phytocannabinoid cannabidiol on experimental colon cancer. *J Mol Med (Berl)* 2012 Aug: 90(8), 925–34.

37. Preet, A., R. K. Ganju, and J. E. Groopman. Delta9-Tetrahydrocannabinol inhibits epithelial growth factor-induced lung cancer cell migration in vitro as well as its growth and metastasis in vivo. *Oncogene* 2008 Jan 10: 27(3), 339–46.

38. Thomas, A. A., L. P. Wallner, V. P. Quinn, et al. Association between cannabis use and the risk of bladder cancer: results from the California Men's Health Study. *Urology* 2015 Feb: 85(2), 388–92.

39. Abuhasira, R., L. B. Schleider, R. Mechoulam, and V. Novack. Epidemiological characteristics, safety and efficacy of medical cannabis in the elderly. *Eur J Intern Med*. 2018 Mar: 49, 44–50.

40. Bargnes, V. H., P. B. Hart, S. Gupta, and L. Mechtler. Safety and Efficacy of Medical Cannabis in Elderly Patients: A Retrospective Review in a Neurological Outpatient Setting. American Academy of Neurology (AAN) 2019 Annual Meeting: Abstract P4.1-014. Presented May 8, 2019.

Chapter 5:

When to Consider Medical Cannabis

As we have seen from the previous chapters, medical cannabis has been used for centuries, just as other plants have been used as medicines for a very long time. We have a system in our body that was here hundreds of millions of years before the marijuana plant even existed called the endocannabinoid system (ECS). The ECS is designed to help regulate a variety of important systems in our body, including pain, hunger, and inflammation. Not only is this system important for normal, everyday function, but research has also shown that certain common conditions may be a result of deficiencies of our own endocannabinoids. We also learned that the marijuana plant contains phytocannabinoids that can act on the endocannabinoid system, leading to many health benefits in certain disease states. While research is limited due to restrictive federal regulations, we have seen that there is a substantial amount of research that does support the use of medical cannabis, especially in the areas of nausea, chronic pain, and muscle spasms. While there is still a stigma against using marijuana as a medicine, thirty-three states (and counting) and the District of Columbia have now legalized medical marijuana, and a network of dispensaries has been set up in these states so that qualifying patients can register and get certified to use medical cannabis legally to treat their medical conditions.

Thus, with the evidence and availability of medical cannabis, when should patients consider medical cannabis as a treatment of their condition? There are two philosophies or ways to think about this, which are not necessarily mutually exclusive.

The first is to consider medical cannabis when all else has failed. This is what I most commonly see when I certify patients. Modern medicine has given use some amazing breakthroughs. Despite some skepticism of the pharmaceutical industry in recent days, they have given us many great products that have changed people's lives. Many of these products are now available over-the-counter and/or available as a generic. When I was a medical student, patients contracting HIV were essentially given a death sentence, and having a blood clot was a seven-day admission in the hospital. Now, patients with HIV can lead normal and healthy lives with one pill a day, and blood clots can be treated with a pill, in many cases without even spending one day in the hospital. Prescription medicines, because of their funding and regulation, are also backed by a tremendous amount of research. Thus, given these benefits, patients should certainly consider conventional, prescription-based treatment for their conditions as initial therapy.

However, there is a limit to what prescription medicines can do. They do not work for everyone. In addition, they often have side effects that can be worse than the condition being treated. Narcotics are an excellent example. For patients in acute pain, such as a severe injury or immediately after surgery, narcotic medications can be wonder drugs and are usually safe and effective. However, for patients with chronic pain, narcotics lose their effectiveness, and patients suffer with side effects such as constipation and nausea. In addition, because of their addictive nature, many patients with chronic pain will get addicted to their narcotic medications. I have seen many chronic pain patients who are suffering from pain despite taking narcotics regularly and also suffering from side effects. In addition, narcotics not only have a high risk for addiction, but also have a low threshold for causing death. Hundreds of patients die each day from opioid overdoses. Thus, when prescription medications are tried and either don't work or cause intolerable side effects, or (as in the case of narcotics) are dangerous, alternatives such as cannabis should be considered.

A second approach would be to consider medical cannabis for certain conditions as a first-line therapy. This may be appropriate when the current initial treatments are not as safe or not as effective as cannabis. Sleep may be a good example to consider. Insomnia is quite common and associated with stress or actual medical mental health conditions like anxiety or depression. Over-the-counter preparations like diphenhydramine are often used by patients before even consulting a doctor. While diphenhydramine is relatively safe, it usually makes people groggy the next day and can cause side effects, especially for men with urinary issues from enlarged prostates. While older prescription medicines like barbiturates are no longer used due to safety and concerns of addition, the newer sedative hypnotics like Ambien (zolpidem) are commonly prescribed. These medications are effective and relatively safe. I have used them successfully in hundreds of patients. However, in addition to not working in every patient as well as causing some sedation the next morning, zolpidem is associated with some uncommon but serious and unusual side effects, such as sleepwalking or raiding the kitchen without realizing it. There have been reports of people driving while still technically sleeping while taking zolpidem. Again, these reports are rare but concerning. Cannabis is a natural product that is effective for sleep, does not usually cause morning sleepiness, and does not have any unusual side effects. In addition, unlike prescription or even over-the-counter medications, marijuana does not usually interfere with other medications. One common group of patients that suffer from insomnia are the elderly, who are also more susceptible to side effects and take multiple medications where interactions can be a concern. Thus, for an elderly patient with insomnia, rather than start with a medicine like zolpidem, which most physicians would likely choose, a better option might be to start with medical cannabis, which should be just as effective, and probably even safer.

Whether or not you are considering medical cannabis as a last resort, or a safer/natural alternative to prescription medications, deciding if medical cannabis is right for you can be challenging. You should certainly discuss this with your physician, but be advised that they may not be supportive. As a physician, my role is to provide patients with the best available evidence to help them make appropriate choices about their health. In some cases, this is pretty easy (e.g., stopping smoking, eating healthy foods, taking antibiotics for strep throat infections). In other cases, it can be more of a challenge when data is conflicting, such as prostate cancer screening and treatment. In regard to medical cannabis, because of the restrictive federal regulations, research is limited. While I firmly believe that there is enough research to suggest medical cannabis for treating patients, many physicians will be uncomfortable making such a recommendation with the data currently available. So I do recommend discussing this with your physician, but you should be aware that she may not be sympathetic nor well versed in the research (as this was not taught in medical school nor published in many of the commonly read medical journals).

In considering whether medical cannabis is right for you, you are going to need to be your own advocate, which means doing research on your own. My hope is that this book will provide you with enough information to help you make an educated decision, as well as a few resources that you can use if you need more information. Also, as we will see later in the book, in states that have legalized medical marijuana, dispensaries have been set up to obtain these products. The staff at the dispensaries have a wealth of knowledge and information and can also be of great help. Finally, while there is valuable information on the internet, proceed with caution. Just like any topic, there is also a lot of misinformation and anecdotal reports.

Part B:

Using CBD
and CBD Oil

Chapter 6:

Using CBD and CBD Oil

The marijuana or cannabis plant has over one hundred different biologically active compounds that can affect your body. There are several cannabinoids, or compounds in the plant (phytocannabinoids), that interact with our own endocannabinoid system to produce a variety of healing effects. While there are multiple cannabinoids in the cannabis plant, the two main cannabinoids are THC and CBD. THC (tetrahydrocannabinol) is the psychoactive component in marijuana that at increased doses can get patients "high" and make them sleepy. Cannabidiol or CBD is the nonpsychoactive component: it will not make you sleepy or "high." Due to the entourage effect, THC and CBD usually work very well when used together. However, CBD on its own also has important medicinal effects, particularly in regard to anti-inflammatory and antianxiety properties. While CBD can be extracted from marijuana, it can also be obtained from another plant source called hemp. Technically, marijuana and hemp are really the same plant. They are both scientifically classified as *Cannabis sativa*. While both marijuana and hemp have cannabinoids and terpenes, hemp has virtually no THC. Essentially, hemp is a cannabis plant that has only trace amounts of THC (0.3%, by definition), and because of this, hemp is essentially legal everywhere in the United States. Because of this fact, CBD products have become readily available for purchase in a variety of places, including independent pharmacies, organic food stores, chain retailers like Bed Bath & Beyond, and even gas stations. However, unlike medical cannabis, which is highly regulated in the states where it is medicinally legal, hemp-based CBD is not yet regulated by the FDA, which causes a great number of challenges for patients and consumers in terms of quality and safety. For the purposes of this chapter, I will use the term CBD generically, and not distinguish between marijuana-based CBD and hemp-based CBD. However, there is theoretically no difference between the two. Again, both are cannabis plants, but hemp is strain that is very low in THC. CBD from both hemp and marijuana affect the body in exactly the same way, but much of the research on CBD comes from marijuana-derived CBD. There is very little research on hemp-based CBD.

History of Hemp-Based CBD

The hemp plant has been used for centuries and continues to be used today for a variety of purposes, including food, paper, and textiles, as well as extracting it for its medicinal properties. Texts dating back to 2737 BC indicate that hemp extract was used as a medicine in China. In ancient Greece, hemp plants were found at burial sites, suggesting an important role in daily life. Hemp was cultivated in England to make clothes and building materials, and European settlers brought industrial hemp to North America in the seventeenth century.

In the 1840s, Irish physician William Brooke O'Shaughnessy published a paper based on his work in India, stating that hemp and cannabis could be used for a variety of medical purposes. It was not until 1940 that Dr. Roger Adams discovered CBD at the University of Illinois, though its structure was not delineated until many years later. Even though CBD was discovered more than two decades before THC, research has focused much more on THC. While most research has been focused on marijuana (THC combined with CBD), interest grew in the medicinal benefits of nonpsychoactive CBD from hemp. In 2013, CNN aired a documentary about medical cannabis titled *Weed*, produced by Dr. Sanjay Gupta. The documentary featured the story of Charlotte Figi, a three-year-old girl who was diagnosed with Dravet syndrome, a rare genetic condition causing intractable seizures. Multiple medications hadn't helped Charlotte, but a strain of cannabis that was very low in THC, but high in CBD, finally did. Charlotte's Web, named after Ms. Figi, is a popular hemp-based CBD product used today. In June 2018, the US Food and Drug Administration approved Epidiolex, a CBD-only purified oral solution derived from marijuana for the treatment of Dravet syndrome and Lennox-Gastaut syndrome, another rare seizure disorder in children.

How Does CBD Work?

The endocannabinoid system is biological system that exists in humans and animals and regulates several bodily functions. While the body makes its own cannabinoids (endocannabinoids), principally anandamide and 2-AG, plant-derived cannabinoids (phytocannabinoids) can also affect this system. The human body has two main cannabinoid receptors: CB1 and CB2. These cannabinoid receptors are scattered throughout the body in places like the brain and nervous tissue (CB1), as well as some organs and the immune system (CB2). Both anandamide and THC act primarily by stimulating the CB receptors. In contrast, CBD has very little effect on the CB receptors, and in fact, CBD decreases the activity of cannabinoids like anandamide and THC at the CB receptor.[1] This explains why CBD can mitigate some of the side effects (getting high) of THC. CBD has effects on other receptors as well. CBD stimulates the serotonin 5-HT1A receptor, which might explain why it is helpful in anxiety and nausea.[2, 3, 4] Other receptors CBD interacts with in the body include adenosine and glycine receptors, which can explain CBD's role in reducing inflammation and pain.[5, 6] In addition to interacting with other receptors, it can inhibit or block the uptake of neurotransmitters. Neurotransmitters such as serotonin, dopamine, and norepinephrine are chemical messengers that work on the brain and the nerves and affect our thoughts and actions. CBD's effect on these neurotransmitters is another way in which it can be effective in anxiety and pain.

Types of Hemp-Based CBD

Until recently, hemp has been grown and processed in a limited number of states, including California, Colorado, Kentucky, Oregon, and Tennessee. However, at the end of 2018, the passage of the US Farm Bill allowed industrial hemp to be grown anywhere in the United States. There are many parts to the hemp plant that have different purposes. For example, fibers from the hemp plant can be used in textiles. One area of confusion are hemp seeds, which can be made into an oil. Hemp seed oil can be used as a food, and may have benefits for the skin, but it contains no CBD. Only the leaves and flowers of the hemp plant contain cannabinoids, including CBD. All hemp-based products are very low in THC, but contain other cannabinoids in small amounts such as cannabigerol (CBG) and cannabinol (CBN), as well as other terpenes. Hemp-based CBD oil generally comes in three varieties: full spectrum (full plant extract), broad spectrum, and isolate (also called purified).

Full-spectrum hemp oil is made from the plant's flowers, leaves, stems, and seeds. Using an extraction method, processors of the hemp plant create an oil that contains cannabinoids, flavonoids, and terpenes from the full plant, including trace amounts of THC. Because some people are concerned about THC, especially regarding drug testing, processors have been able to isolate just CBD in a pure form (isolate), which contains only CBD. Interestingly, research has shown that even in small amounts, the various cannabinoids and terpenes tend to have a greater effect when used in combination rather than alone, called the "entourage effect." Research has also shown that increasing the dose of full-spectrum CBD, but not isolate CBD, causes increased benefits without side effects. Thus, full-spectrum CBD tends to work better than CBD isolate.[7] Another available option is broad-spectrum CBD (also called phytocannabinoid rich or PCR), which eliminates only the THC, but adds back the other important cannabinoids and terpenes. In general, I recommend full-spectrum CBD oil when using this medicinally, as it can take full benefit of the entourage effect having the most amount of cannabinoids (including trace amounts of THC) and terpenes.

Diseases Treated with CBD

SEIZURE DISORDER

As mentioned, the story of Charlotte Figi exemplifies CBD's use in seizure disorder. The purified-marijuana-based Epidiolex was approved by the FDA to treat the severe forms of seizures seen in Dravet syndrome and Lennox-Gastaut syndrome. In order to be approved by the FDA, the manufacturer had to prove the benefit of CBD/Epidiolex in several rigorously done, randomized clinical trials.[8] While the dosing of Epidiolex is quite high (up to 20 mg/kg a day, or 1,200 mg a day for a typical adult), other studies have shown that using a more phytocannabinoid-rich hemp-based CBD preparation can decrease seizures in much lower doses.[9]

ANXIETY AND DEPRESSION

Many daily antianxiety medications work by decreasing the uptake of certain neurotransmitters, which is just one way in which CBD may help with anxiety symptoms. While there are a few small studies that show that high-dose CBD might reduce acute anxiety before a stressful event, such as public speaking,[10] CBD has better evidence if taken on a daily basis, at lower doses (around 25 mg daily) to reduce general anxiety.[11] Most patients with PTSD in one small study saw significant improvement in symptoms when taking daily CBD.[12] There is less evidence for depression, but research on both animals and humans indicate that CBD may have antidepressant properties as well.[13, 14]

ARTHRITIS

While THC tends to be better for pain in general, CBD appears to be effective particularly on pain caused by inflammation. One of the most common diseases of pain caused by inflammation is osteoarthritis. Osteoarthritis is the wear and tear of bones caused by overuse and aging. This process leads to inflammation, which causes pain. CBD may have direct effects on inflammatory cells or may modulate the effects of certain pain receptors in the spinal cord.[15] While human studies are lacking, in an experimental model using rats, CBD was able to prevent pain caused by joint inflammation.[16]

CANCER

While most studies are related to cancer have been performed on animals or in test tubes, there is some promising research that cannabinoids like THC and CBD may have a role in cancer treatment. THC in particular can be useful in both treating the symptoms of cancer (bone pain from cancer spread) and the side effects of treatment (nausea from chemotherapy). However, CBD and THC may actually help treat and even prevent cancer. There are several research studies showing that cannabinoids can increase the rate at which cancer cells die, as well as prevent cancer cells from spreading.[17] There is even some preliminary data in human patients with cancer who had a positive response in reduction in tumor growth when given CBD for at least six months.[18]

CBD Side Effects

While CBD is considered generally safe without any psychoactive effects, no substance given to humans is completely without any potential harmful effects. While CBD is not sedating for most patients, some patients have told me that it relaxes them and therefore makes them somewhat sleepy. These patients will actually take their CBD at night to help them sleep. The best evidence to determine CBD side effects is to look at the Epidiolex studies,[19] which is the FDA-approved agent for seizures in children. Because this was scientific study (randomized trial) comparing it to a placebo, one can make more accurate determinations of side effects or adverse events. According to the studies, the most common adverse reactions that occurred in the Epidiolex-treated patients (which happened at least in 10% of treated patients and more than placebo) were somnolence; decreased appetite; diarrhea; transaminase elevations; fatigue, malaise, and asthenia; rash; insomnia, sleep disorder, and poor quality sleep; and infections. It is important to note that the doses used in these trials were much higher than usually used (about forty times more) by patients. Of all of these, transaminase, or liver enzyme elevations, are probably the most concerning. It is important to note that in the trials, the patients who were most likely to get liver enzyme elevations were also taking other seizure medications.

The other potential issue with CBD is interactions with other medications. However, even in the Epidiolex trials, in which high doses were used, the FDA did not note any drugs that CBD could not be taken with. Rather, it noted that some medications might need to be adjusted if taking (in this case, very high doses of) CBD. There are certain enzymes that break down pharmaceuticals in the body. When you block or inhibit these enzymes, the drug levels may rise, and when you induce or stimulate these enzymes, the drugs that they metabolize may fall, and you might need to increase the dose of the prescription medication. CBD inhibits the drug-metabolizing enzymes CYP3A4 and CYP2D6 and can therefore increase levels of drugs metabolized by these isoenzymes. Thus, a dose reduction could be required in drugs metabolized by these enzymes. These medications include certain antibiotics (macrolides like azithromycin), some blood pressure medications (calcium channel blockers), some anxiety medicines (benzodiazepines), and certain medications taken for HIV (antiretroviral).

CBD for Pets

While veterinary use of marijuana and CBD is beyond the scope of this book (and my expertise), in discussing CBD, I feel it is important to point out that CBD is becoming more and more popular with veterinarians in treating common ailments for pets. Because hemp-based CBD is legal everywhere, it is easy for veterinarians to recommend CBD for their patients, and many of the companies selling CBD products to humans are also selling similar products for pets. While dosages are slightly different based on the weight of various animals compared to humans, the use of CBD is almost identical. As mentioned, CBD is particularly good for inflammation (such as that seen with arthritis) and anxiety. Similar to humans, these issues are common with pets. While evidence for CBD is even more limited for pets than humans, there is at least one randomized controlled trial[20] that showed that dogs with arthritis who received CBD oil (2 mg/kg versus a placebo twice a day) showed improvement in activity and pain.

How to Use CBD and CBD Oil

Because hemp-based CBD is legal everywhere in the United States, it is popping up everywhere. In addition to CBD oil, CBD is now available in food, drinks, soaps, creams, and bath bombs. In April 2019, Carl's Jr. became the first fast food chain to sell a CBD-infused hamburger when it offered its Denver customers a "Rocky Mountain High Cheeseburger Delight," though just for one day. Research on CBD—and hemp-based CBD in particular—is limited. While there are several areas where research suggests CBD may be helpful, such as anxiety and inflammation, most of the research and experience regarding CBD comes from ingesting CBD oil, either directly in a liquid (tincture) or in a pill form (oil capsule). There is no scientific evidence supporting any benefit to topical CBD (creams) and no scientific evidence to support the use of CBD in bath salts or bath bombs. Any claim on these uses is based on anecdotal evidence. While topical CBD has been reported to help with joint and muscle pain, as well as skin conditions, it is unlikely to be effective for muscle and joint pain because the CBD cannot penetrate deep enough through the skin to affect those underlying tissues. Conversely, skin conditions could have a benefit from topical CBD, since the CBD does not need to penetrate as deeply. I have many patients who have tried topical CBD creams. Most say that they noticed little to no difference. However, a few noticed some relief from joint and muscle pain. In addition, many topical CBD products come with other ingredients that may have an effect. For example, many CBD creams are just a combination of methyl salicylate and/or menthol (the ingredients in Bengay) plus CBD. So is it the CBD that is helping, or the other ingredients? Thus, while there is likely little harm in trying

CBD in any of these formulations (especially topicals, which are now sold at mainstream pharmacies), in general, I only recommend CBD oil, which can be used as a tincture, where it is placed under the tongue, or in oil capsules, via which it is swallowed.

There is a potential advantage over tinctures in some circumstances, as when it is placed under the tongue, the CBD can be absorbed more readily into the bloodstream (and act faster) as opposed to swallowing oil capsules, which must first be broken down in the stomach and then absorbed into the bloodstream through the intestines. As far as dosage, unlike THC, which should be slowly titrated until effects are achieved without side effects, higher dosages can be initiated right away, as there are few to no side effects with CBD. Most studies seem to show benefits when CBD is taken at a 15 mg daily dose or higher. I generally recommend a daily dose (either all at once or divided during the day) of 25 mg to 33 mg hemp-based CBD oil, either in tincture (dropper) or oil-capsule formulation.

The Regulatory Problem of Hemp-Based CBD and How to Obtain Quality CBD Oil

As mentioned, CBD is a cannabinoid found in both hemp and marijuana, but unlike marijuana, which is federally illegal and only medically legal in certain states, hemp, because it has virtually no THC (the cannabinoid that can make you high) is legal everywhere in the United States. The advantage of the legal status of hemp-based CBD is that it is a readily available agent that can be easily purchased at prices that are usually much lower than marijuana-based CBD. This is particularly true of cannabis-based CBD sold at the medical dispensaries in states where marijuana is medically legal, since the regulatory process that ensures both purity and safety of the CBD products sold in the dispensaries is expensive to maintain. However, the one problem with hemp-based CBD is that it is not currently regulated by the FDA. The Food and Drug Administration (FDA), which not only regulates prescription medications, but also food, vitamins, and supplements, has not decided whether or not hemp-based CBD should be regulated like a supplement/vitamin or regulated like a prescription drug. On May 31, 2019, the FDA held a public hearing at which opinions from all sides were heard. While the FDA has committed to making a decision sometime soon, currently CBD stands in a regulatory no-man's-land. Big chains like CVS and GNC have decided not to sell CBD oil (though they are selling CBD cream, as this is regulated differently) until things are sorted out. However, small retail stores (including even gas stations) as well as a multitude of online websites sell unregulated CBD. In the past, the FDA analyzed some of the CBD oil products that were sold online. In most cases, the amount of CBD listed in these products was not accurate, and in some cases, the CBD products sold online had absolutely no CBD in them at all! For these reasons, since 2016, the FDA has sent warning letters to these companies, though no other action has been taken.[21]

While this doesn't mean that hemp-based CBD is dangerous, it does mean that if you are going to use hemp-based CBD preparations, you must take time to ensure the quality and accuracy of the product, which may take some extra research on your part. There are several things to look out for. The company should be reputable and have a good track record, as anyone can create a fancy website now. They should also use good farming practices, including using non-GMO industrial hemp grown without pesticides. However, probably the most important factor to look at before purchasing or using any hemp-based CBD product is that it must be independently verified for quality, purity, and accuracy by an outside, third-party, qualified lab to determine the exact contents of what you will be taking. You should not purchase or use any hemp-based CBD if you cannot verify the exact ingredients (including what is not in it, such as pesticides and other chemicals) by an independent (i.e., not owned by the company making the CBD) laboratory. There are only about a dozen companies in the United States that make high-quality, third-party independently verified full-spectrum CBD oil. There are many more that are not independently verified, so choose carefully.

Chapter 6 Notes

1. Morales, P., et al. Allosteric modulators of the CB1 cannabinoid receptor: a structural update review. *Cannabis and Cannabinoid Research* 2016: 1(1), 22–30.

2. Russo, E. B., et al. Agonistic properties of cannabidiol at 5-HT1a receptors. *Neurochemical research* 2005: 30(8), 1037–1043.

3. Resstel, L. B. M., et al. 5-HT1A receptors are involved in the cannabidiol-induced attenuation of behavioural and cardiovascular responses to acute restraint stress in rats. *British journal of pharmacology* 2009: 156(1), 181–188.

4. Limebeer, C. L., D. E. Litt, and L. A. Parker. Effect of 5-HT 3 antagonists and a 5-HT 1A agonist on fluoxetine-induced conditioned gaping reactions in rats. *Psychopharmacology* 2009: 203(4), 763.

5. Mecha, M., A. Feliú, P. M. Iñigo, L. Mestre, F. J. Carrillo-Salinas, and C. Guaza. Cannabidiol provides long-lasting protection against the deleterious effects of inflammation in a viral model of multiple sclerosis: a role for A2A receptors. *Neurobiol Dis* 2013: 59, 141–150.

6. Xiong, Wei, et al. Cannabinoids suppress inflammatory and neuropathic pain by targeting α3 glycine receptors. *Journal of Experimental Medicine* 2012: 209(6), 1121–1134.

7. Gallily, R., Y. Zhannah, et al. Overcoming the Bell-Shaped Dose-Response of Cannabidiol by Using Cannabis Extract Enriched in Cannabidiol. *Pharmacology & Pharmacy* 2015: 6, 75–8.

8. Devinsky, O., H. Cross, et al. Trial of Cannabidiol for Drug-Resistant Seizures in the Dravet Syndrome. *N Engl J Med* 2017: 376, 2011–2020.

9. Sulak, D., R. Saneto, and B. Goldstein. The current status of artisanal cannabis for the treatment of epilepsy in the United States. *Epilepsy & Behavior* 2017: 70, 328–333.

10. Bergamaschi, M. M., R. H. Queiroz, et al. Cannabidiol reduces the anxiety induced by simulated public speaking in treatment-naïve social phobia patients. *Neuropsychopharmacology* 2011 May: 36(6), 1219–26.

11. Shannon, S., et al. Cannabidiol in Anxiety and Sleep: A Large Case Series. *Perm J* 2019: 23, 18–41.

12. Elms, L., S. Shannon, S. Hughes, N. Lewis. Cannabidiol in the Treatment of Post-Traumatic Stress Disorder: A Case Series. *Journal of Alternative & Complementary Medicine* 2019 Apr: 25(4), 392–397.

13. Hill, M. N., and B. B. Gorzalka. The endocannabinoid system and the treatment of mood and anxiety disorders. *CNS Neurol Disord Drug Targets* 2009 Dec: 8(6), 451–8.

14. de Mello Schier, A. R., N. P. de Oliveira Ribeiro, et al. Antidepressant-like and anxiolytic-like effects of cannabidiol: a chemical compound of Cannabis sativa. *CNS Neurol Disord Drug Targets* 2014: 13(6), 953–60.

15. Xiong, W., C. Tanxing, et al. Cannabinoids suppress inflammatory and neuropathic pain by targeting α3 glycine receptors. *J Exp Med* 2012 Jun 4: 209(6), 1121–1134.

16. Philpott, H. T., M. O'Brien, and J. J. McDougall. Attenuation of early phase inflammation by cannabidiol prevents pain and nerve damage in rat osteoarthritis. *Pain* 2017: 158(12), 2442–2451.

17. Massi, P., et al. Cannabidiol as potential anticancer drug. *British journal of clinical pharmacology* 2013: 75(2), 303–312.

18. Kenyon, J., W. Liu, and A. Dalgleish. Report of objective clinical responses of cancer patients to pharmaceutical-grade synthetic cannabidiol. *Anticancer research* 2018: 38(10), 5831–5835.

19. https://www.accessdata.fda.gov/drugsatfda_docs/label/2018/210365lbl.pdf

20. Gamble, L., J. M. Boesch, C. W. Frye, et al. Pharmacokinetics, Safety, and Clinical Efficacy of Cannabidiol Treatment in Osteoarthritic Dogs. *Vet Sci* 23 July 2018.

21. https://www.fda.gov/news-events/public-health-focus/warning-letters-and-test-results-cannabidiol-related-products, accessed 10/6/2019.

Part C:

Using Medical Cannabis and CBD

Chapter 7:

General Advice for Using Medical Cannabis and CBD

If you are reading this chapter, then you have at least decided that medical cannabis and/or CBD might help you or a loved one with a particular medical condition. However, the amount of information (or misinformation) on this topic can be confusing and overwhelming. In addition, even if you have done your research and have determined that medical cannabis or CBD might be a good option, how to obtain medical cannabis and use it appropriately and effectively can be even more daunting. To help you or a loved one, this section and the next is designed to guide you step by step; the last section of this book gives very specific recommendations about how you can use medical cannabis and CBD for specific medical conditions or diseases. In this section, we will focus on how to use medical marijuana and CBD safely and effectively. This includes choosing the correct strain of cannabis (Chapter 8); using the correct type of cannabis product (e.g., edible, topical), known as its formulation (Chapter 9); making sure you take the right dose (Chapter 10); and finally, considering any potential side effects or drug interactions (Chapter 11). The next section of the book (Part D) goes over in detail how to obtain medical cannabis and CBD, reviewing how to register and get certified, as well as what to expect when going into a medical dispensary to purchase medical cannabis. However, before diving into these details, here is some general advice for using medical cannabis and/or CBD.

Why Use Medical Cannabis and/or CBD?

Marijuana is a plant that has been used as a medicine for thousands of years. In fact, many of the medicines we use today to treat conditions like emphysema, heart disease, and pain are derived from plants. Medical cannabis has been scientifically proven to treat a number of specific conditions such as nausea, muscle spasms, and chronic pain. It can also be very useful in a variety of common conditions such as anxiety, depression, and insomnia. Unlike some prescription medications, medical cannabis is safe, nonaddictive, and has few to no side effects or interactions with other medications. Cannabis works because it contains multiple compounds called cannabinoids that can affect your body. The reason they work with your body is that the human body has a natural endocannabinoid system and makes its own cannabinoids (endocannabinoids), which act with cannabinoid receptors in the body. Thus, using medical cannabis and/or CBD is a natural way to affect the body's own natural regulatory system.

While there have been many advancements in medicine, including the development of lifesaving drugs; medications don't always work, and even if they do, they are sometimes accompanied by intolerable side effects. Another advantage of using medical cannabis and/or CBD is that, if used the correct way, is not only effective, but can have very few side effects. Many of the patients I have treated with medical cannabis had used prescription medications that were either not working or had too many side effects. One of the most common conditions I treat with medical cannabis is pain, including patients who are on narcotics. The current opioid crisis was caused by many factors that are beyond the scope of this book, but a few important relevant factors are that pain is common, there are few effective treatments, and while opioids can be very effective, they are highly addictive and can be fatal if taken incorrectly. In contrast, medical cannabis has little to no addictive properties and is nonlethal. If you take too much cannabis, it can make you very sick or very high, but it will not kill you.

Recreational Marijuana versus Medical Cannabis

Because marijuana is used both recreationally and medicinally, even in states where medical marijuana is legal, there is still a stigma regarding using it as a medicine. While the marijuana plant can be smoked and used as a recreational drug, medical marijuana—more properly referred to as *medical cannabis,* since cannabis is the scientific name—when taken correctly should not get patients "high," and does not need to be smoked. As previously stated, plants have been used as medicine for thousands of years. In addition, the poppy seed plant has been used to make or synthesize medicines (opioids like oxycodone and codeine), which have been used as medicine effectively for some time, even though it is also used to make recreational narcotic drugs like heroin. A major difference, as mentioned, between opioids and cannabinoids is that the former is addictive and can be lethal, while the latter is not.

Many of the patients whom I certify for medical cannabis come to me having some success trying recreational marijuana as a medicine and come to me to get certified to use cannabis legally and safely. Thus, it is important to distinguish between using recreational marijuana medicinally and using medical cannabis. In addition to legal factors (as of this writing, recreational marijuana is legal in nine states and the District of Columbia), the difference between recreational marijuana and medicinal cannabis is how the quality and safety of the products are regulated. Recreational marijuana generally has no regulation in terms of quality and safety. You essentially must trust your grower, dealer, or supplier. In contrast, medical cannabis sold at state-regulated dispensaries is highly regulated by the state with strict criteria and standards for growers, processors, and dispensaries to maintain. This allows you as a patient to know exactly what you are getting and that there are no other chemicals or pesticides in the product. It also has the specifics as far as the strain you are taking, the terpene content, and the amounts or percentages of cannabinoids. In contrast, with recreational marijuana, you likely will not even know what strain you are getting, let alone its terpene profile or percent THC. Thus, medicinal cannabis can be used safely as a medicine; whereas recreational marijuana has medicinal effects, there are concerns when using as a medicine. Finally, while there are multiple formulations (smoking, edibles) for both recreational marijuana and medicinal cannabis, medicinal cannabis sold at state-regulated dispensaries generally have a larger variety of formulations, whereas recreation marijuana is more often smoked.

Marijuana versus Hemp-Based CBD

CBD is a cannabinoid that, unlike THC, has no psychoactive properties; it cannot make you "high" or sleepy. While marijuana has both CBD and THC, the related plant hemp has virtually no THC, so it is legal in most states and can be purchased online (and in some stores) without going through any certification process. Thus, hemp-based CBD is usually easier to get and cheaper than marijuana-derived CBD. There is theoretically no difference between marijuana-based CBD and hemp-based CBD, and in fact they are technically the same plant. However, because hemp-based CBD is not regulated by the FDA, you must be very careful that you are getting a high-quality, full-spectrum, third-party-verified product. In general, while I generally recommend patients use both CBD and THC to treat a variety of medical conditions, in order for them to save some money, I will often recommend that they use hemp-based CBD purchased online or in some stores, along with medical cannabis that they purchase in a dispensary. Since finding good-quality, third-party-verified, hemp-based CBD can be challenging, I recently started offering hemp-based CBD to patients seen in my office.

The Most Effective Ways to Use Medical Cannabis and CBD

When using medical cannabis, two things that are most important are choosing the correct strains of cannabis and using the right formulation. There are different strains of cannabis that have different effects for different conditions. In regard to formulation, while there many ways or formulations to take medical cannabis, including smoking or ingesting the actual cannabis leaves (known as "bud" or "flower"), I do not recommend smoking, both because it is not good for your health, and because it is very hard to dose a puff. I also generally do not recommend ingesting medical cannabis (e.g., using the bud or flower to make your own brownies or other kinds of food), because it is also difficult to dose, and ingesting too much cannabis could lead to side effects. The four ways to take medical cannabis that I recommend for most patients are tinctures, pills or edibles, vape, and topicals. The two main factors in determining the right formulation is onset of action (how quickly it works) and duration (how long it lasts). For something acute, like a migraine headache, something that works in minutes is necessary, while help with sleeping through the night requires something that lasts a long time. Thus, the best ways to use medical cannabis and CBD is to not smoke recreational marijuana, but rather to obtain medical cannabis from a state-regulated dispensary, often combining this with high-quality hemp-based CBD that is verified by an independent third party; choose the correct strains of cannabis for your particular ailment; and then use the right formulations of cannabis products, specifically not smoking the flower, to achieve the desired effects. In addition, there are a few other important things to consider:

Multiple formulations are usually needed. When I make specific recommendations for my patients, I often give them three to five different products to use, with instructions on how to use and adjust the dose for each one. Multiple products are often needed because people have different symptoms that require different treatments. For example, patients with chronic pain usually have pain all the time, as well as severe breakthrough pain. Thus, I might recommend an edible that takes a while to start working but lasts six to eight hours. However, they will also need something fast acting, like a vape for breakthrough pain.

Start low and go slow. One of the very nice features of cannabis is that you can usually achieve the desired medical benefit (pain relief, anxiety relief, et cetera) without getting high or sleepy. The key to achieving this goal is by starting with very low doses of THC and slowly adjusting the dose each time, monitoring the effects with each dose. By starting low and slowly adjusting or titrating medical cannabis, most patients can get relief without adverse effects.

Everyone's a little bit different. Another reason to go slow is that everyone reacts to cannabis slightly differently. In addition to some people being more or less sensitive to THC, different strains can affect people differently. For example, indica strains are supposed to make people relaxed and sleepy. However, there are some patients that have the opposite effect and do better with a sativa strain.

You must be patient. Because multiple formulations are usually needed, because it is best to start at a low dose and slowly titrate the medication, and because individuals may have a slightly different reaction to each product, successful use of medical cannabis does not happen overnight. You need to be patient and persistent. I have seen many patients with whom it took several trials of a variety of different products over several weeks before they were able to achieve benefit. While medical cannabis may not be right for everyone, of the thousand-plus patients I have certified for medical cannabis, the vast majority achieve some benefit from medical cannabis.

Chapter 8:

Strains

Overview

As discussed in the first section of this book, cannabis is a plant that contains a variety of different substances that can affect the body, and thus have medicinal properties. Cannabinoids in plants (phytocannabinoids), like THC and CBD, interact with CB receptors in the human body affecting the endocannabinoid system (ECS) to produce effects ranging from pain, mood, and inflammation. Other components of the plant also have effects, including substances called terpenes, which, similar to other plants, fruits, and spices, give cannabis its smell and flavor. Terpenes themselves have a variety of medicinal properties and can affect the body through a variety of mechanisms. Finally, all of these components work together synergistically, in what is known as the entourage effect, to produce the overall effect on the human body and thus ultimately how cannabis is used as a medicine.

There are multiple strains of marijuana plants, which each have different amounts of CBD, THC, as well as different types and amounts of terpenes (often called the strain's "terpene profile"). It is the combination of all of these factors that give each strain its unique medicinal properties, and make one strain of cannabis better for one condition or another.

Indicas and Sativas

Evaluating the different strains of cannabis plants is partially an exercise in botany. The cannabis plant belongs to the genus of flowering plants in the *Cannabaceae* family. There are a number of species within this genus, which is sometimes disputed. However, one convention is to label the cannabis plant as *Cannabis sativa*. Hemp is also *Cannabis sativa* and is differentiated from marijuana primarily by the limited of amount of THC (less than 0.3%, by definition). There are a number of strains of the *Cannabis sativa* plant, with a variety of different properties.

While there are a number of ways that cannabis strains are divided or group, in general, strains are labeled as either into indica or sativa strains. While the effects of the different strains are more determined by their terpene profiles and amounts and ratios of THC and CBD, there are some differentiating properties of indica and sativa strains. Indica strains tend to be more relaxing and sedating. They have been used to help with insomnia and anxiety, as well as helping with muscle spasms and tremors. Sativa strains tend to be more alerting. They have been found to increase appetite and help with pain, and have been used for depression.

In addition to the indica and sativa strains, growers of the cannabis plant have developed hybrid strains that are a mix of both indica and sativa. Hybrid mixes of both strains allow some strains to have a variety of properties that may be effective in certain situations—for example, to alleviate anxiety without being too sedating. Furthermore, hybrid strains can be dominant in either indica or sativa, or a balance of both. Thus, strains can be categorized as indica, sativa, balanced hybrid, indica-predominant hybrid, or sativa-predominant hybrid.

Common Strains

There are hundreds of different cannabis strains, and new ones continue to be developed and gain popularity. The availability of different strains will likely depend on what is commonly grown in your state. In addition, there may be a significant difference between the cannabinoid content and terpene profile in the same strain grown in one state compared to another. Since there is no significant clinical research that truly can determine which strain is best for which condition, most of the available information is anecdotal. Internet searches of cannabis strains for specific medical conditions are likely to yield a variety of different and sometimes conflicting recommendations. One orthopedic surgeon, Dr. Frank D'Ambrosio, who treats patients with medical cannabis in California and is a medical cannabis advocate, surveyed 4,276 of his patients to find out which strains they used and for which of the thirty-nine different conditions they were treating.[1] Thus, while it would be impossible to review every cannabis strain and its effects on a variety of different medical condition, below is a list of some of the most common strains and conditions for which they are effective. This list has been developed based on a variety of resources, including Dr. D'Ambrosio's work, reputable websites, discussions with cannabis experts, and experiences from my own patients. Of note, the actual names of the different strains of cannabis are still derived from their recreational use. Thus, many of the names do not sound like traditional medications, and in fact can be humorous and sometimes overtly offensive. While this can take some getting used to, especially for more conservative medical patients who have never used recreational marijuana, keep in mind that the medicinal properties of these strains are both very real and effective, and should be taken seriously.

Sativas

JACK HERER

Jack Herer is a sativa-dominant strain, with an average amount of THC. Jack Herer also has a terpene called terpinolene, which has a floral aroma and can be found in apples, lilacs, and nutmeg. This strain was named for the late marijuana activist Jack Herer, who wrote the 1985 pro-cannabis book, *The Emperor Wears No Clothes*. Jack Herer is felt to be less potent than other strains and thus is considered a very good choice for patients who are new to medical marijuana. It is not very sedating and therefore good for daytime use. It has been particularly useful in anxiety disorders and painful conditions such fibromyalgia.

ACAPULCO GOLD

Acapulco Gold gets its name from its origins in Acapulco, Mexico. It is a sativa strain with caryophyllene as its predominant terpene. It is known to be energizing and elevates mood, which is why it can be useful to treat fatigue and depression. It also has some benefit in reducing nausea.

Sativa-Dominant Hybrids

BLUE DREAM

Blue dream is a sativa-dominant hybrid, rich in myrcene and pinene, with some caryophyllene. It has relaxing properties, but due to its sativa predominance (and despite its high THC content), it does not cause substantial sedation and can be slightly invigorating. Given the lack of sedative effects, Blue Dream is popular for daytime users who want to be fully functional. It is particularly good for depression but can also be used for pain and nausea.

SOUR DIESEL

Sour Diesel is another sativa-dominant hybrid strain. It is different in that its predominant terpene is caryophyllene and limonene, with some myrcene. Sour diesel is also nonsedating and much more energizing. Thus, it is particularly popular for use in depression and can provide a productive calm with a boost of energy for those patients who are stressed. It can also be used for pain relief, such as headache and fatigue.

Balanced Hybrids

GIRL SCOUT COOKIES (GSC)

Girl Scout Cookies, also referred to as GSC, is a balanced hybrid, with caryophyllene and limonene as its predominant terpenes, plus a little humulene. It has a high THC concentration with little CBD. It can be used for severe pain, nausea, and loss of appetite.

WHITE WIDOW

White Widow is another balanced hybrid containing an average THC concentration, along with myrcene, caryophyllene, and a little limonene in its terpene profile. Its attributes are mood improvement and energy, but without sedation; thus, it is most commonly used for depression and fatigue.

Indica-Predominant Hybrids

SKYWALKER OG

Skywalker OG is an indica-predominant hybrid strain. Given its high amounts of THC (20%–25%), it can be very sedating and thus is excellent for insomnia. It has a very rich terpene profile, containing alpha-Pinene, as well as many others. It is also a powerful painkiller, especially pain secondary to injury or muscle cramps. It causes relaxation; thus, it is good for anxiety and stress.

GORILLA GLUE

Gorilla Glue (Gorilla Glue #4) is also an indica-predominant hybrid strain, with a little more sativa than Skywalker OG, but an even higher amount of THC (25%–30%). Thus, this is a strain that probably shouldn't be used in patients new to medical cannabis. With a terpene profile including linalool, humulene, and caryophyllene; it has an aroma that is said to be somewhat like chocolate. While powerful, especially for conditions such as chronic pain, insomnia, and muscle spasms, it is also more likely to cause a "high."

Indicas

GRANDDADDY PURPLE (GDP)

Granddaddy Purple (or GDP) is an indica strain, with myrcene and caryophyllene as its predominant terpenes, and an average amount

(17%) of THC. Like most indicas, it is relaxing and sedating, and thus is useful in anxiety and insomnia. It is also good for pain, increasing appetite, and relieving muscle spasms.

Northern Lights

Northern Lights is a pure indica strain with a slightly lower than average amount of THC. Similar to GDP, it has myrcene and caryophyllene as its predominant terpenes, with a little bit of limonene. Northern lights is also a relaxing, sleep-inducing strain that can simultaneously elevate mood. It is used for insomnia, pain relief, depression, and anxiety. It's also known for its mood-lifting effects.

Chapter 8 Notes

1.   D'Ambrosio, F. Report: Can Cannabis Reduce
      the Need for Addictive Pharmaceuticals? Accessed
      online February 5th, 2018: https://doctorfrank.com/
      study-2018-can-cannabis-replace-addictive-pharmaceuticals/.

Chapter 9:

Formulations

Overview

The last chapter discussed differences in the types of cannabis strains and how different strains are used for different conditions. However, even if you have chosen the right strain, you need to decide how you are going to consume that strain. While strains of marijuana plants have been smoked, either recreationally or medicinally, for centuries, there are a variety of methods to get the beneficial effects of marijuana's cannabinoids and terpenes into your body. The term I use for describing the various types of medical cannabis products is "formulation." This is the "form" of the strain/cannabinoids you will be using and, in most cases, must be formulated in a certain way so that all the biologically active ingredients are able to be absorbed into your body. In addition, using the raw plant isn't really formulated, so the term "formulation" better applies to anything that is not pure plant. Having multiple formulations allows patients to use medicinal cannabis in a variety of ways without having to smoke marijuana or prepare the plant in some other fashion. While there are a variety of formulations, I will focus mostly on those that I recommend and describe a few others that I don't recommend in general but might be used in certain circumstances. I will not be able to describe all possible formulations of medical cannabis, as they are so many and they are evolving every day.

Flower

SMOKING FLOWER

There are many names used for smoking marijuana, either for recreational or medicinal purposes. "Weed" and "pot" usually refer to recreational use of the marijuana plant. While the marijuana plant might be best recognized by its characteristic leaves, the leaves of the plant are not what is normally smoked. Rather, it is the flowers and/or buds of the plant that have the most trichomes, which are small algae-like projections that have the highest concentrations of cannabinoids. Thus, when referring to the consumption of the raw marijuana plant, even for medicinal purposes, marijuana is often referred to as "bud" or "flower." Flower can be used without smoking, but in general, when consumers or patients refer to using *flower*, they generally mean that they are smoking it.

There are many purists who insist that flower is the best way to use cannabis medicinally. While I disagree, it is important to understand their argument. In fact, it is the raw, natural, unprocessed flower that has the most amounts of terpenes, flavonoids, and cannabinoids compared to other cannabis formulations. When formulating a cannabis product that is not smoked, such as a pill or cream, some of these vital components can be lost, theoretically making nonflower products less effective.

While this in fact may be true, in my opinion, many of the theoretical benefits of using the whole plant are likely offset by the dangers of smoking. To explain, it may be helpful to look at tobacco. Nicotine cigarettes have three harmful ingredients. The first is the nicotine itself, which is highly addictive and can cause increases in heart rate and blood pressure. The second are the chemical additives put into cigarettes by the tobacco companies to increase shelf life, improve taste, et cetera. These chemicals themselves can be toxic. However, even raw, dried-out tobacco leaves devoid of chemical additives would still be harmful when smoked. Smoke is by definition incomplete combustion (if everything combusted, you wouldn't see anything after the substance burned). Much of the small particulate matter in smoke is carbon. This carbon or ash, whether from tobacco or cannabis, can be harmful to the lungs. Smoking tobacco or cannabis also produces carbon monoxide, which is not only bad for the environment but also decreases the body's ability to get oxygen from air when breathing. Smoke from both tobacco and cannabis has thousands of ingredients, some of which have been determined to cause cancer. While both recreational and medicinal users may use water pipes (bongs) to filter the smoke, most of the harmful ingredients still remain, even after this filtration. Thus, for all of these reasons, I never recommend that patients smoke flower to get their medicinal cannabis.

USING FLOWER WITHOUT SMOKING

With the benefits from the whole plant and the dangers from smoking it, it is not surprising that people have looked for ways to use flower without smoking it. While there are likely a number of creative ways of doing this, the most common ways of using flower without smoking are ingestion and vaporizing.

There are many ways to ingest cannabis flower, such as baking the flower into brownies. While patients can eat the brownies, the term *edibles* (which I will discuss below) usually describes formulated or manufactured tablets or gummies, and not foods like brownies or cookies (though some processors manufacture formulated versions of foods, such as chocolates or cookies, that can function like edibles). While ingestion is a much safer way to use flower than smoking, I also do not generally recommend ingestion. The problem is that since we are using flower as a medicine, a proper and precise dose (in my opinion) is very important. Just like when you are baking cookies, you can't be sure about the exact numbers of chocolate chips in a given chocolate chip cookie; the amount of cannabis in each brownie or cookie might be too much, causing unwanted side effects, or may be too little and thus not effective. There are many recipes on the internet for making cannabis butter, teas, or other ingestibles. However, in my opinion, cannabis is a serious medicine, and just like I would not want my regular patients making their own blood pressure or cholesterol medicine, I don't recommend ingestion as a safe form of cannabis use.

Vaporizing cannabis is different from using vapes (which I will discuss below). Flower is placed in a device called a vaporizer (which come in a variety of shapes and sizes), that heats cannabis flower to between 330–370°F, which causes the active ingredients in the flower to evaporate into vapor without causing combustion (which happens at 451°F) of the plant material, theoretically eliminating the harmful parts of smoking. Essentially, vaporizing flower cooks or boils the flower to extract the medicinal products, as opposed to smoking, which does the same thing but causes the harmful by-products of combustion: ash and carbon monoxide. While vaporizing dry flower seems to be much safer than smoking flower, safety studies haven't been performed, and it's not clear that all toxins are eliminated. More importantly the process of preparing and storing the flower properly, as well as some of the challenges of selecting and using the right vaporizer, can be complex. For these reasons, especially for new patients, I usually recommend non-flower vaping (described below) over dry flower vaporizing. However, vaporizing dry flower correctly can be a very reasonable option for medicinal cannabis use.

Recommended Formulations

TINCTURES

A tincture by definition is a medicine that is made by dissolving a drug in alcohol and usually refers to plant-based medicines. While cannabis tinctures aren't necessarily dissolved using alcohol, in the medical cannabis world, tinctures are liquids containing cannabinoids that usually come in a bottle with a dropper and are administered to patients by placing those drops under their tongues. By placing drops under the tongue, as opposed to swallowing the liquid, the drops sit in the mouth for a few minutes while the medicine is absorbed directly into the bloodstream. Your mouth has a lot of blood vessels, so delivering medicines under the tongue can be both efficient and fast. If the dose is large and thus not entirely absorbed, any remaining medicine is swallowed. In fact, tinctures can be swallowed whole, usually by placing drops in another liquid and swallowing, but this negates some the benefits of a faster onset of action if placed under the tongue.

Some tinctures are made the old-fashioned way by using alcohol to extract the essential ingredients from the cannabis. Medical cannabis processors that make tinctures for dispensaries may use other methods, which may not contain all of the original cannabinoids and terpenes from the whole plant. Rather, they will extract the cannabinoids from the plant and add some of the terpenes back later in the process. Processors might also add other components back to a tincture, such as botanicals and flavoring. For example, a manufacturer might add some melatonin to an indica-predominant tincture to better improve sleep.

While you can find instructions to make your own tinctures on the internet, I don't generally recommend this for patients, since there is no way to know the exact dose. By contrast, tinctures purchased from a dispensary usually have exact milligrams of THC and CBD and come in predictable ratios, like 2:1. Tinctures often work quite well for patients who are new to medical marijuana because they are generally easy to dose, easy to start at a very small dose and slowly increase the dose, and easy to consume. If taken under the tongue, tinctures usually take about thirty to forty-five minutes to work, but last in the body for four to six hours.

EDIBLES

While you can ingest flower baked into a brownie, edibles generally refer to a processed cannabis product that can be chewed and/or swallowed. Edibles come in the form of oil capsules, mints, pills (which can be chewed or must be swallowed), and gummies (sometimes referred to as troches). Edibles are very easy to consume and often have flavoring like mint or fruit that makes their taste pleasurable. Edibles are not as easy to start with very low doses as tinctures. While a 5 mg pill can be cut into a 2.5 mg dose, cutting pills in quarters or smaller can cause issues with accurate dosing. Edibles are usually more processed than other forms of cannabis. This gives edibles consistent dosing reliability (a 5 mg pill should have 5 mg of cannabinoid in it), but this likely comes at a cost of having some of the valuable cannabinoids, terpenes, and flavonoids from the whole plant processed out of the final product. Like tinctures, some of these ingredients may be added back in the end. Edibles also tend to have a greater amount of THC per dose than tinctures. There are edible gummies that have 20 mg per chew or higher. Thus, edibles may be the best way for patients who require higher doses of THC to consume cannabis. Edibles can take a bit longer to work, usually forty-five to sixty minutes, because they must first pass through the gut before being absorbed into the bloodstream. However, they also last much longer (six to eight hours), which is good for symptoms that occur all throughout the day or throughout the night.

VAPE

As above, vaporizing cannabis generally refers to using a vaporizer to heat dry flower in order to inhale the vaporized products without smoking. Vape, on the other hand, generally refers to inhaling the extracted oil from the cannabis plant using a vaping device. Cannabis processors use a variety of methods to extract all of the whole-plant components from the cannabis into a concentrated liquid or oil (known as "concentrate"). The concentrate is then put into a cartridge, and that cartridge is placed into a device called a "vape" or "vape pen." The vape pen is a battery-operated device that heats the oil concentrate so that it is vaporized and can then be inhaled. There are also nicotine vapes, known as electronic cigarettes or e-cigarettes (Juul, Blue), that use a similar process. Recently there has been serious concern about off-brand or black-market nicotine vapes that have caused severe lung damage, leading to serious illnesses and even death. The CDC has determined that most of these serious cases were due to a vitamin-E derivative that black-market vape manufacturers of e-cigarettes were using to dilute the amount of nicotine in their products. The advantage of using medical cannabis purchased from a state-sanctioned dispensary is that it is highly regulated. You know exactly what you are getting (the percent of THC, the terpene profile, the date the plant was harvested), and possibly more importantly, what you are not getting (pesticides and additives like vitamin-E derivatives). Thus, cannabis vapes should be safe to use if they are obtained from a state-sanctioned medical cannabis dispensary. In some states, both medical cannabis and recreational marijuana is legal and sold in dispensaries. While the problems with vape occurred in illegal electronic cigarettes, I would not necessarily trust vapes sold at a legal recreational marijuana dispensary.

One advantage of cannabis vape is that because it is often a full extract from cannabis flower, vape has the full benefits of all the cannabinoids and terpenes from the whole plant without having to be smoked. In fact, depending on where you live, almost any cannabis flower strain can be found in a vape. Vape also works very quickly (seconds to minutes), which is very beneficial for acute and severe conditions. However, vape also doesn't last very long (an hour or so), meaning that any sedation or other effects will disappear quickly, so you can get back to your day. However, it may not be the best options for a symptom that occurs constantly, such as chronic pain. Vapes generally come as either a reusable device and a disposable cartridge, or in an entirely prefilled, disposable vape "pen," which can be discarded when the oil or concentrate is used up. I generally recommend first-time users start with disposable vape pens for their ease of use and convenience. While vape is inhaled, there are no adverse health effects like one would get from smoking. Using vape may seem a bit odd for patients new to medical cannabis, but it is quite easy to use.

TOPICAL

Topical formulations of medical cannabis, such as salves or balms, can be very effective for localized pain. Despite some of these formulations having a high amount of THC, because they are applied to the skin, very little is absorbed in the bloodstream, and thus topical formulations generally have no psychoactive properties. Balms or creams only last a few hours and thus should be applied regularly. However, they are an excellent option because of their low side effect profile. Topical formulations are particularly good for pain when it occurs on a specific area of the body, such as low-back pain. However, when patients have pain all over the body, topical formulations may not be the best way to go.

OTHER FORMULATIONS

As mentioned, I generally do not recommend flower, either smoking it or ingesting it (though vaporizing flower may be a reasonable option). I also don't recommend making your own tinctures or other formulations for accuracy concerns and ease of use. My preferred formulations are tinctures, edibles, vapes, and topicals that are made by a reputable processor and sold in a state-sanctioned medical cannabis dispensary. I will generally recommend more than one formulation at a time. For example, an insomnia patient who has trouble both falling asleep and staying asleep might benefit from both a vape to help them fall asleep as well as an edible to help keep them asleep. However, while most patients can achieve excellent results without smoking, just using these four formulations, sometimes this isn't enough. There are a variety of other formulations, and because newer ones are popping up each day, they are too numerous to mention here. However, below are a few alternative nonflower options, which I don't generally recommend, especially for first-time users. However, they may have a role in a very select number of patients, so I will discuss briefly for completeness.

OTHER CONCENTRATES

A concentrate is any product that is derived from cannabis flower that has been processed into a more concentrated form. Technically, most of the formulations mentioned, including some tinctures and edibles, are concentrates. However, *concentrate* usually refers to a much more concentrated form of cannabis. The concentrated oil used in a vape cartridge for vaping is a concentrate, and sometimes vapes are referred to as concentrate. Since there are many prefilled vape pens with concentrated oils that come in practically every strain, I recommend vape as a preferred way to use cannabis. However, there are a few other concentrates that may be appropriate for some patients, though a bit more challenging to use.

Shatter and wax are two types of concentrates made from flower. There are a variety of ways to extract all of the cannabinoids, terpenes, and other important components from cannabis flower. Solvents such as butane and carbon dioxide can create highly potent extracts. Shatter is an extract that is clear and hard, with a glasslike appearance. Wax is another concentrate that is opaque and soft, essentially a thicker, pliable oil. Similar to vaping, shatter and wax must be heated so that their oils are vaporized and can be inhaled by the user. In order to do this, the wax or shatter is placed in a device called a dab rig. Here the wax or shatter is placed on a ceramic, glass, or titanium surface called a nail, and heated up with a small torch. Dabbing is commonly used in recreational cannabis. Because of the challenges of consistent doses, the high concentrations of THC in dabbing shatter and wax, and other dangers of dabbing, including starting a fire, I don't generally recommend this technique. Vaping is a safer and more consistent way to inhale concentrated cannabis oil.

Rick Simpson oil is also known as RSO. It is a highly concentrated cannabis oil developed by Rick Simpson, a Canadian cannabis activist who created the product to treat his own skin cancer. Since RSO is highly concentrated, it can contain up to 90% THC, which is much higher than the typical vape pen. RSO is usually dispensed out of a syringe. Because of the high concentration and potency, RSO is usually ingested by taking a drop the size of a grain of rice, either on placed on your finger or a small piece of food like a cracker and swallowed. Given the high potency and that fact that the size of one grain of rice might be vary with each use, RSO doses can be inconsistent from one dose to the next. In addition, the high potency increases the risk for overdosing and causing side effects. RSO should not be used by a novice. However, for patients that require a high amount of THC, RSO might be the most efficient and cost-effective way to consume potent cannabis.

OTHER TOPICALS

A topical preparation is anything that you apply to your skin. I highly recommend topicals such as balms or salves because they can be highly effective and are generally not absorbed by the skin into the bloodstream and therefore have no side effects. However, there are preparations that can be applied to the skin that are absorbed by the bloodstream. These topicals are known as transdermals. Transdermals are typically administered in a patch that is applied to an area on the skin where there are a lot of blood vessels for the cannabinoids to be absorbed. The wrist is a common place to use a transdermal. Transdermal patches may take some time to work, but likely last the longest of any other cannabis formulation, for up to twelve hours. Gel pens are another form of transdermal preparation. Gel is released from the pen when applied to the skin. It is applied to similar areas as a transdermal patch. Gel pens can work more quickly than patches and last up to six hours. Transdermal patches and pens can be a fabulous option for patients. The reason I do not typically recommend these products is that they tend to be very expensive. One patch, which is often one day's dose, can cost more than $20, compared to a 5 mg THC edible mint, where a dozen mints might cost the same amount.

Chapter 10:

Dosing and Titration

Overview

Even if you have determined the correct strain of medical cannabis to use (indica, sativa, predominant hybrid, et cetera) as well as the correct formulation to use (tincture, edible, et cetera), you still need to determine the correct dosing, as well has how to titrate the dose. Dose is the amount of medication you take. If you are taking 10 mg of Lipitor once a day to treat cholesterol, the "strain" is Lipitor, the formulation is tablet, and the dose is 10 mg once a day. *Titration* means slowly increasing the dose of a medication.

Dosing of cannabis can sometimes be complex. First, certain formulations like vapes and topicals have a variable amount of cannabis in them depending on how big of a puff you take or how much cream you use. In addition, when it comes to edibles, pills, and tinctures, the way current products are labeled make it difficult to determine the exact dose. For example, many hemp CBD products are commonly sold and labeled as milligrams of CBD per bottle and not milligrams per dose or dropperful.

Many, if not most, prescription medications are taken without titration. However, some medications are titrated (i.e., started at a low dose and increased to a higher dose to minimize side effects). Doctors will also titrate a medication to achieve a specific outcome. For example, insulin is often titrated in diabetics until a target sugar level is achieved. If you start the insulin dose too high, the blood sugar will get too low and patients will feel light-headed and can even pass out. If the insulin level is too low, the sugar will not be controlled. Thus, titrating medical cannabis is generally means starting at a low dose of medication, and slowly increasing the dose until the desired effect is achieved without having any unwanted side effects, such as feeling sleepy or "high."

While medical cannabis has both THC and CBD, and both have effects on the body, only the THC is the psychoactive component. Thus, titrating the dose of medical cannabis generally means titrating the effects of the THC. There is one major important concept for medical cannabis that is true across all dosing titration schedules, regardless of the strain or formulation: *start low, go slow.* This means starting at a low enough dose of THC where patients might feel some effects but at a low enough dose where side effects are very unlikely to occur. When starting at such a low dose, it is not uncommon for a patient to feel no effect at all. However, patients can then slowly increase the dose until they feel some improvement in symptoms without any side effects. Going slow is also important because the body gradually gets sensitized to cannabis. The first use of cannabis will stimulate synthesis of new cannabinoid receptors in the body, such that the same dose on day 3 may have more of an effect than the dose on day 1.

CBD-to-THC Ratios

CBD and THC have both similar effects (antianxiety, antinausea, pain relief) and opposite effects (THC increases appetite; CBD reduces appetite). Using THC and CBD together have benefits not only due to the entourage effect (different cannabinoids and other compounds like terpenes working synergistically to achieve a desired effect), but also because CBD seems to counteract some of the undesirable effects of THC, such as feeling sedation or feeling intoxicated or "high." Thus, I believe that regardless of which formulations patients use, there should always be at least some combination of both THC and CBD. Even for patients taking hemp-based CBD alone, I recommend full-spectrum products because they have trace amounts of THC.

Many products contain both CBD and THC, so when considering which products to use as well as the correct dose and titration, it is important to know the CBD-to-THC ratio. For flower and vape, ratios are not generally listed for specific strains, but rather percent of CBD and THC are reported. For example, Catatonic is a pure hybrid strain high in myrcene and pinene, which is often used for pain. Catatonic is considered to have a low concentration of THC, with 3%–7% THC and 6%–10% CBD, and thus is less sedating than other strains. So, while ratios are not typically reported for specific strains, often due to the variability between strains, one could consider Catatonic a 2:1 strain, meaning that there is about double the amount of CBD than THC. For tinctures and edibles/pills that are more processed, the exact amount of both CBD and THC are usually known, so ratios are often listed. Depending on where you live and the dispensary you use, tinctures and edibles/pills can come in a wide variety of ratios, from 20:1 to 1:1. When a ratio is listed, CBD is usually but not always first, so read labels carefully. A 2:1 tincture or edible/pill means that for every 2 mg of CBD, there is also 1 mg of THC. Vireo, a cannabis company that has dispensaries and makes products in ten different states, has product lines of capsules and tinctures that come in the following ratios: 1:19, 1:6, 1:1, 6:1, 19:1. Thus, a 1:19 tincture is mostly THC, and a 19:1 capsule is mostly CBD.

Choosing the right ratio can be tricky, and there not a great deal of evidence regarding which one is best. The largest body of clinical research on humans in regards to ratio is with a balanced or 1:1 ratio. Nabiximols is a pharmaceutical-grade cannabis pill available in Europe that has a 1:1 ratio. It has been studied in many patients, mostly those with chronic pain and multiple sclerosis. At this ratio, the pain-relieving effects of THC are very good, with few adverse effects. Dose and cost can also be an important factor. For example, THC is a strong reliever of pain. Patients wanting pain relief without sedation might choose a high CBD-to-THC ratio product, such as a 10:1 tincture. A 15 ml bottle of such a tincture might sell for about $70. Half of a dropperful will have about 10 mg of CBD and almost 1 mg of THC. Assuming a patient needs one dropperful three times a day to control their pain, the $70 bottle will only last five days ($420 for a month's supply). However, a 1:1 tincture might only cost only $40 for four times the amount of THC. So a thirty-day supply of the THC would only be $80, or one-fifth the cost. While this would be substantially less CBD, the CBD can be obtained at a much more affordable price by combining with hemp-based CBD. A thirty-day supply of 30 mg capsules of high-quality hemp-based CBD can be obtained for around $100 or less, retail. Thus, given the research available for balanced CBD:THC ratio products, the higher cost of high CBD:THC ratio products, and the lower cost of hemp-based CBD, I generally recommend patients combine a low CBD:THC ratio product (tincture, pill, edible), such as 1:1 or 2:1, with a higher-dose hemp-based CBD tincture or capsule, rather than using high CBD:THC ratio products (e.g., 10:1, 15:1, 20:1, et cetera).

Dosing and Titration of Specific Medical Cannabis Products

In general, dosing and titration of specific products depend on the formulation of the product and the CBD:THC ratio. As mentioned in the previous chapter, the formulations I usually recommend are creams, edibles or pills, tinctures, and vapes. Other formulations can be titrated in a similar fashion. In general, cream does not need to be titrated, because only minimal amounts are absorbed in the bloodstream. *Dosing* not only refers to the amount of cannabinoids you take, but also how often you will use cannabis during a twenty-four-hour period. The dosing intervals (once a day versus every few hours) depends on the duration of the formulation. The following sections explain how to dose and titrate CBD, vapes, edibles, and tinctures.

DOSING AND TITRATION OF CBD

As mentioned above, I tend to recommend a high-dose CBD product taken in addition to medical cannabis products that contain both THC and CBD. Because CBD has no psychoactive effects, it does not need to be titrated. Thus, separating the CBD not only helps decrease the cost of using medical cannabis, but it also allows patients to maximize the dose of CBD for greatest efficacy. The most benefit from CBD is seen above 15 mg, and for many conditions, 25 to 30 mg is enough to achieve benefit from CBD. Thus, I recommend that patients take a daily dose of 25 to 30 mg of hemp-based CBD in either capsule or tincture formulation, without titration. CBD can be taken once daily or split into twice-daily intervals. Tincture and oil capsules are both good formulations to use. As discussed in the chapter on CBD, it is very important if using hemp-based CBD to ensure that it is high quality and independently verified by a third-party lab.

DOSING AND TITRATION OF VAPE

Dosing and titration occur somewhat simultaneously, as there is no way to know the exact milligrams of THC when vaping because everyone's "puff" is going to be a little different. First, choose the strain of your vape based on the desired effect needed (e.g., indica-predominant strain with high myrcene content) as well percentage of THC. In general, 13% THC or less is considered to be a light THC strain, 14%–20% THC is considered to be a medium or average THC strain, and 20% THC or greater is considered to be a high-THC strain. Once you have chosen the right strain and THC concentration, start with one small puff. You should feel the effects of the vape within two minutes. If you don't feel anything, you can take another puff. Continue taking small puffs every few minutes until you feel something. Once you feel some effects, then hold on that amount with each dose for the next few doses. You may find enhanced effects at the same number of puffs with subsequent doses. Once you feel confident of the effects on your body with the least number of puffs it takes to feel something, you can then titrate vape both by slowing increasing the number of puffs or increasing the volume of puff you take (i.e., start with a small puff but increase to a bigger puff). Eventually, you will determine the number of puffs it takes to achieve the desired effect (e.g., reduce anxiety, reduce pain) without feeling sleepy or high. For most patients, this lies somewhere between one and three puffs. Also, you may vary your dose based on time of day and desired/undesired effects. For example, one small puff during the day may be enough to relieve anxiety without making you sleepy, so you can get your job done at work. However, you may choose to take two puffs when you get home since sedation may be less of a concern by then, and three puffs before bedtime to help make you sleepy. The effects of the vape usually last for about an hour; thus, some patients may need to vape several times a day.

DOSING AND TITRATION OF EDIBLES OR PILLS

The advantage of pills and/or edibles are that they last a long time, approximately six to eight hours. Thus, dosing intervals can usually be much less frequent (e.g., three times a day). The disadvantage of pills and/or edibles are that they take a long time to start working (i.e., up to an hour). This is very important in terms of dosing, and starting low in particular, because too high of a dose of pills/edibles will take a while to leave the system. One of the reasons I do not recommend using flower as an edible (such as using flower to make cookies or brownies) is that it is too difficult to start with a low dose, which can subsequently have long-lasting negative effects. One milligram of THC is usually the lowest dose needed to achieve an effect, so I will generally recommend starting between 1 mg to 2.5mg of THC in an edible two to three times a day. Since sedation is a side effect of THC, edibles can be used for helping patients with insomnia, with a starting dose that is slightly higher if used before bedtime. The milligrams of edibles or pills should be easiest to determine since this is usually indicated clearly on the package. However, this is not always the case, as sometimes the total amount of THC is what is on the label. In that case, divide the number of pills or edibles per package by the total milligrams of THC. So if there is a pack of 100 mg THC with ten edibles, then each edible has 10 mg of THC. Look also for the ratio of CBD:THC. Even for a variety of ratios, the milligrams of CBD and THC are usually labeled on the box of edibles or pills, but not always. For example, one company makes a 2:1 tablet, which is available in a forty-tablet bottle labeled as having 2.5 mg of CBD. Since the pill is 2:1, the amount of THC is 1.25 mg per pill. In this example, the amount of THC is not labeled on the bottle and therefore has to be calculated. So if there is double the amount of CBD to THC, and there is 2.5 mg of CBD, then the amount of THC is half the amount of CBD, or 1.25mg. Since starting low is even more important for edibles, I would recommend starting with no more than one tablet two to three times a day, increasing the dose by a half a tablet (0.625 mg of THC) each day until any effects are noticed. Once any effects are noticed, I would stay on that dose for a few days, and then continue to increase by half a tablet a day until the dose given three times a day achieves the desired effects without any side effects (sedation, feeling "high").

DOSING AND TITRATION OF TINCTURES

Whereas vape works quickly but doesn't last long, and edibles/pills last a long time but take a long time to work, tinctures are a nice in-the-middle solution. They work in about thirty minutes and last about four to six hours, so dosing intervals are about four or more times a day. Tinctures are somewhat trickier to dose because the milligrams per dose are not always obvious on the packaging. Typically, packaging will list the milligrams per bottle, but not much more, so math is often involved. Bottles typically come in 15 ml and 30 ml amounts, so the first step in dosing is to determine the milligrams per milliliter (mg/ml). A 30 ml bottle with 1,000 mg of CBD, has 33.3 mg/ml.

Tinctures are usually delivered by droppers. You drop the tincture under your tongue, let it sit there for a few minutes to absorb, and then swallow the rest. Another complexity to tincture dosing is that droppers are not standardized. However, most droppers are 1 ml droppers, and most drops are one-twentieth of a milliliter, or 20 drops per 1 ml. Thus, in order to determine the dose, you need to know mg per bottle, volume of bottle, and the CBD:THC ratio of the product. For example, there are 2:1 tinctures that contain 200mg of CBD and 100mg of THC in a 15-ml bottle. This means there is 6.7 mg (100 divided by 15) of THC per milliliter or dropperful. At 20 drops per milliliter, 5 drops, or one-quarter of a dropperful, would equate to 1.67 mg THC and 3.33 mg of CBD. As stated above, one milligram of THC is usually the lowest dose needed to achieve an effect, so in the case of this particular tincture, I would start with just 3 to 5 drops every 4 to

6 hours, increasing the dose by 1 to 2 drops at a time, until any effects are noticed. Once effects are noticed, I would recommend staying at that dose for the next few doses or days to ensure the maximal effect is achieved, and then continue to slowly increase (titrate) up the dose, again one drop at a time, until the desired effects are achieved without any side effects (sedation, feeling "high").

Chapter 11:

Safety and Side Effects

Overview

While medical cannabis can be used as a very effective medication with a limited number of side effects and interactions with other medications, no substance is completely safe. Many consider marijuana safer than prescription medications because it is "natural." While being from nature does have many benefits, not everything in nature is non-harmful. Arsenic, snake venom, botulinum toxin, and mercury are all natural substances. Thus, when considering the risks of medical marijuana, one must look at it from a number of different perspectives. First and foremost is lethality. In addition, because medical cannabis is a Schedule I drug, which by definition means it is addictive, the addictive properties of medical cannabis must also be examined. Because medical cannabis is still federally illegal, it is also important to look at it from a societal lens, including marijuana being labeled as a "gateway drug," as well as the potential risks of traffic accidents and fatalities due to increased availability. Another safety issue for any medication is risk of interactions with other medications. Finally, we need to consider adverse effects, or "side effects," of medical cannabis. We have spent considerable time discussing euphoria, or feeling "high," as well as sedation, which are the most common potential unwanted effects; however, there are others to consider. The remainder of this chapter examines each of these issues closely. Hopefully, you will be convinced that despite some adverse effects and safety issues, which occur with any medication, that the benefits of medical cannabis far outweigh any negatives, and thus should be readily available to all patients.

Medical Cannabis: Lethality and Addiction

One way to consider lethality and addiction of medical cannabis is how it compares to other commonly used substances, both legal and illicit, as well as recreational and medicinal. Figure 1 (below)[1] plots dependence potential, or how addictive a drug is, against lethality, defined as the active-to-lethal dose ratio. Dependence ranges from low to high, with marijuana being moderately low in dependence or addiction, and nicotine being considered high. The active dose is the amount of substance you need to have an effect, and the lethal dose is the amount of the substance that is likely to kill you. Alcohol, for example, is considered to have a relatively high active-to-lethal dose ratio of 0.1, which means that one dose (let's say one beer or glass of wine) is enough to have an effect, but ten drinks all at once can possibly kill you. While is it rare for humans to die of alcohol ingestion, likely because it is uncommon to ingest a case of beer or three bottles of wine all at once, there are certainly reports of college students dying from being hazed and attempting stunts like this. From the graph you can see that marijuana has a fairly low dependence rate (on par with caffeine) as well as a low risk of lethality (lower than most other substances). Thus, from an addiction or lethality standpoint, it can be argued that cannabis, and certainly medical cannabis, is much safer than even coffee or alcohol. In addition, it is clear from this standpoint that narcotics, including prescription medications, are clearly far more dangerous. This table also helps to explain why the opioid crisis facing this country is such a problem. Patients become highly addicted to their chronic opioid pain medications, and if they accidentally take too much—even just one extra pain pill—it can easily lead to death. One of the reasons that cannabis is thought to be far less dangerous than opioids is because research shows that there are very few cannabinoid receptors on the brain stem, while there are many opioid receptors on the brain stem. The brain stem is the nonthinking part of our brain that is responsible for keeping us alive. It controls breathing and regulates heart rate. Overdoses of narcotics, doses that are in fact not much higher than the therapeutic doses used to treat conditions, can cause suppression of respiration and ultimately death. Taking too much cannabis might make you sleepy, sick, or high, but it will not kill you. No one has ever died from cannabis.

Figure 1: Active/Lethal Dose Ratio and Dependence Potential of Psychoactive Drugs

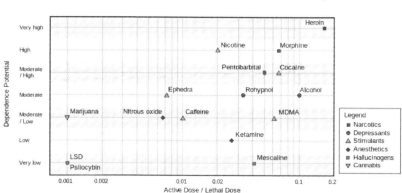

Medical Cannabis Leading to Substance Abuse

One concern regarding use of recreational marijuana, and thus medical cannabis as well, is that it will lead to abuse of other substances. There has been a persistent notion that cannabis might be a "gateway" drug to other illicit substances. As discussed in Chapter 4 (Medical Cannabis Research), in 2017, the National Academies of Sciences, Engineering, and Medicine reviewed all the available research on medical cannabis and published their findings in a document titled "Health Effects of Cannabis and Cannabinoids: Current State of Evidence and Recommendations for Research."[2] As mentioned in Chapter 4, there were three areas where there was compelling research supporting use of medical cannabis for nausea related to chemotherapy, chronic pain, and muscle spasms related to MS. However, they also reviewed studies looking at cannabis and its relationship to other substances of abuse. They made the following conclusions:

1. There is limited evidence of a statistical association between cannabis use and the initiation of tobacco use.
2. There is limited evidence of a statistical association between cannabis use and changes in the rates and use patterns of other licit and illicit substances.
3. There is moderate evidence of a statistical association between cannabis use and the development of substance dependence and/or a substance abuse disorder for substances including, alcohol, tobacco, and other illicit drugs.

In other words, there is very little evidence to support recreational marijuana use as a drug that leads to the initiation of other drugs. However, there is an association with marijuana use and dependence on other drugs. This should not be surprising since marijuana is also used as a recreational drug, and people who will develop substance abuse of other recreational drugs may in fact also use marijuana. In other words, the research shows that while substance abusers may use marijuana, marijuana does not appear to lead to abuse of other substances (i.e., it is not a "gateway drug").

In terms of marijuana being "addictive," it is important to define what that means. According to the American Society of Addiction Medicine, "addiction is a treatable, chronic medical disease involving complex interactions among brain circuits, genetics, the environment, and an individual's life experiences. People with addiction use substances or engage in behaviors that become compulsive and often continue despite harmful consequences."[3] In other words, people who are addicted have a compulsive need to use substances despite harmful consequences. Part of the compulsion is when the body becomes physically dependent on a substance, then not taking the substance causes withdrawal symptoms. There is limited data on substance abuse for recreational marijuana, ranging between 9% to 30%.[4] There is also limited data on dependence seen with recreational marijuana use, which is fairly low, with 9% becoming dependent (comparted to 15% of alcohol users or 32% of nicotine users).[5] There is very little information on substance use disorder with medical cannabis, which one would expect to be lower, given the way in which it is used, as well as the generally lower amounts of THC. However, in the clinical trials for the European prescription medical cannabis nabiximols (Sativex—not available in the United States), there were no reports of substance abuse in over thirty thousand patient years of usage.[6] The bottom line is that substance abuse and dependence can occur with recreational marijuana, but is usually lower than other substances, and while there is limited research on substance abuse with medical cannabis, it is most likely very low, with no occurrences in a series of studies with a prescription version available in Europe.

Medical Cannabis and Traffic Safety

While it is illegal to drive with either recreational or medicinal cannabis, people may still do this, and thus, there are concerns about legalizing marijuana and the impact on public safety. Interestingly, while cannabis may impair driver's reaction time and lane position, unlike alcohol, people are usually aware of their impairment and can use judgment to avoid driving while impaired.[7] While there is no breath test similar to alcohol, in which a police officer on the scene could determine levels of cannabis, if impairment is suspected, anyone can be pulled over and tested roadside for signs of intoxication (e.g., told to walk in a straight line). In terms of actual fatalities and crashes, the data is mixed. In some early studies, there seemed to be an increase in traffic accidents in states introducing cannabis legalization. However, one large study[8] that looked at Colorado, Washington, and Oregon, as well as their neighboring states, found that while that in the year those three states legalized recreational cannabis, traffic related fatalities increased by one per one million citizens (a low rate) in the legalizing and neighboring states, the fatality rates went back down to normal a year later. While the effect of cannabis on driving, accidents, and fatalities should be monitored, its impact seems far less than other legal substances, particularly alcohol.

Side Effects of Medical Cannabis

While I generally tell patients that medical cannabis is safe and effective with little to no side effects and few drug interactions, there is no medication that works 100% of the time, nor is there any medication that has absolutely no unwanted effects, and medical cannabis is no different. However, determining the side effects of medical cannabis is challenging for several reasons. First, medical cannabis is used differently than recreational cannabis (e.g., at much lower doses), so while the effects of both are often conflated, the comparison is not fair. I have seen many patients who stated that they "tried pot in college" and didn't like the effects. However, this was likely because they were smoking cannabis and took too large of a dose or "hit." Second, unlike most prescription medications for which a doctor tells you to take one pill a day, medical cannabis should generally be titrated (started with a very low dose to avoid any unwanted effects, and then slowly increased until the desired effect is achieved without any unwanted side effects). For example, if a patient titrates their dose a bit too high and feels a little dizzy, but then backs down on the dose and finds that they can get pain relief without getting dizzy after lowering the dose, is dizziness really a side effect of medical cannabis? Finally, some of the "side effects" are not necessarily harmful or unwanted. Medical cannabis can cause sedation. This is unwanted during the day but can be desired at night. Also, while I instruct my patients to titrate their dose to achieve the desired effect without feeling "high," mild euphoria may be desired for some patients.

Another reason while discussing side effects with medical cannabis is challenging is because the most scientific way to determine side effects is to compare the agent in question to a placebo, or sugar pill. This is how side effects are determined for prescription medications, but randomized, placebo-controlled trials for medical cannabis are extremely limited. For prescription medications, the FDA has a specific way of classifying side effects, and if you have seen any recent TV commercial for a prescription medication, you are already probably familiar with it.

Contraindications are instances when a medication may not be administered (e.g., "Don't take Viagra if you are using nitrates, as this can cause a severe drop in blood pressure"). The only likely contraindication for cannabis is pregnancy, as THC can affect fetal brain development and has been associated with adverse outcomes such as low birth rate.[9] Even this isn't absolute, because most of the research on cannabis and pregnancy comes from recreational marijuana; however, given the potential risk, I would agree with this contraindication. A common contraindication for prescription medications is allergic reactions, which are sometimes observed in studies. While allergy to cannabis, especially touching or ingesting the plant, is known to exist, reports of true anaphylaxis are exceedingly rare, so it is unlikely that this would be listed as a contraindication.

Warnings and precautions are usually listed together. Warnings are severe side effects that have been reported ("Tell your doctor if you have severe muscle pain when taking Lipitor" or the famous "Erections lasting more than four hours" with Viagra). Precautions are observed or potential risks in certain populations ("Use Zoloft with caution in patients with seizure disorder"). There really aren't any major warnings for cannabis. Paranoia can be experienced with very high doses of cannabis, but actual psychosis is very unlikely. There is one study that showed a very low association with psychosis and heavy cannabis usage in young men (highest risk group) of 1 case in 2,800, but only 1 case in 10,000 in light users.[10] For heavy, long-term users of recreational marijuana, there is a condition that has been reported called cannabinoid hyperemesis syndrome, which patients describe repeated episodes of severe abdominal pain, nausea, and vomiting. Scientists are unclear exactly what causes this, but it usually resolves in several days after stopping cannabis.[11] Since this is most often seen with chronic users of high-THC products that are smoked, it is unclear whether this syndrome applies to medical cannabis. In terms of precautions, medical cannabis can temporarily increase blood pressure and heart rate. While it is unlikely that cannabis use can cause a heart attack or stroke, and the association between the two are quite rare, patients with known cardiovascular risk should probably use cannabis with caution (e.g., low doses of nonsmoked products).

Adverse reaction is the term the FDA uses for side effects. By FDA definition, an adverse reaction is an unwanted effect that happens in more than 2% of patients and occurs more than placebo. One of the reasons that headaches are listed as an adverse effect of almost any prescription medication is because headaches are common, so in a study of a drug where 11% of patients on the medication reported a headache compared to 10% of patients with placebo, this would be reported as an adverse event, when in reality it is more likely just a coincidence. Since there are limited randomized studies that compare medical cannabis to placebo, it is difficult to know the true adverse events. One recent review in the *Journal of the American Medical Association* (*JAMA*) of seventy-nine medical cannabis trials (though not all had a placebo), which included 6,462 patients, found that adverse events included dizziness, dry mouth, nausea, fatigue, somnolence, euphoria, vomiting, disorientation, drowsiness, confusion, loss of balance, and hallucination.[12] Dronabinol (Marinol) is a synthetic form of THC approved by the FDA. In their studies, the most common adverse reactions reported (between 3% and 10%) were abdominal pain, dizziness, euphoria, nausea, paranoid reaction, somnolence, abnormal thinking, and vomiting.[13] However, since this is a synthetic cannabinoid, it is not exactly the same as medical cannabis. Sativex is a prescription not available in the United States that is more like medical cannabis, in that it uses extracts of cannabis in a 1:1 THC to CBD ratio. In their placebo studies,[14] using the FDA's definition, adverse effects included somnolence, dizziness, dry mouth, nausea, vomiting, confusion, feeling abnormal or drunk, constipation, diarrhea, fatigue, decreased appetite, and depression. All of these were fairly low, and the ones that were clearly increased from placebo were somnolence, dizziness, dry mouth, nausea, vomiting, confusion, and feeling abnormal or drunk, which seen as very consistent with the *JAMA* review.

So if there were a TV commercial for medical cannabis, the warnings might read something like this:

"Do not use medical cannabis if you are pregnant or may become pregnant. Do not drive or operate heavy machinery when using medical cannabis. Patients with heart disease and schizophrenia should consult with their doctor before using medical cannabis. Tell your doctor if you have repeated episodes of vomiting when using medical cannabis. The most common side effects of medical cannabis are feeling sleepy, dizziness, dry mouth, nausea, vomiting, or feeling confused, disoriented, or drunk. Tell your doctor about all the medications you are taking, as medical cannabis may have interactions. Ask your doctor if medical cannabis is right for you."

Compared to other prescription medications (and other pharmaceutical TV commercials), while medical cannabis does have some contraindications, warnings, precautions, and adverse reactions, these seem far less serious than many, if not most, prescription medications.

Drug Interactions with Medical Cannabis and CBD

Just like any other prescription medication, medical cannabis and CBD can interact with other medications. It is important to note that interaction is not the same thing as contraindication. While there are interactions that can lead to a contraindication (like nitrates with Viagra/sildenafil as mentioned above), most drug interactions do not lead to restriction of usage, but rather consideration of dose adjustment of one or the other medication. This is because our bodies metabolize (break down) medications using a variety of enzymes, which some medications and cannabinoids share. These enzymes are called cytochrome P450 enzymes (or CYP enzymes) that are important in clearing the body of a variety of compounds, including medications. Certain medications or cannabinoids can induce these CYP enzymes, meaning that drugs metabolized by those CYP enzymes will have blood levels reduced and thus will potentially (but not definitely) be less effective. Similarly, certain medications or cannabinoids can inhibit or block certain CYP enzymes, meaning that drugs metabolized by those CYP enzymes will have increased blood levels and thus will potentially (but not definitely) cause more adverse effects.

Despite all this potential interaction, when these interactions are actually studied, there is actually a low risk of observed clinical effects, though there is limited data on humans.[15] In the Sativex trials (prescription marijuana extract not available in the United States), no clinically significant interactions were seen in humans or animals taking drugs metabolized by these shared CYP enyzmes.[14] A similar lack of clinically important interactions was seen in the Epidiolex studies (FDA-approved marijuana-derived CBD product indicated for seizures), though warnings in the label for potential interactions remain.[16]

THC induces CYP1A2 and therefore can reduce levels of drugs metabolized by CYP1A2. These medications include clozapine, duloxetine, haloperidol, chlorpromazine, olanzapine (used for mental health conditions), naproxen (Aleve), and cyclobenzaprine (a muscle relaxant).

CBD inhibits CYP3A4 and CYP2D6, and can therefore increase levels of drugs metabolized by these isoenzymes. For CYP3A4, these medications include macrolide antibiotics (azithromycin, erythromycin), calcium channel blockers (blood pressure medicines), benzodiazepines (used for anxiety, such alprazolam or Xanax), cyclosporine (an immunosuppressive agent used in cancer), PDE5 inhibitors (like Viagra), antihistamines, antiretroviral medications (used in HIV/AIDS), and some statins (cholesterol lowering medications). For CYP2D6, these medications include SSRIs (antidepressant medication), tricyclic antidepressants, antipsychotics, beta blockers, and opioids.

THC and CBD are both metabolized by CYP enzymes as well; thus, their effectiveness can be possibly affected by medications that induce or inhibit shared CYP enzymes. Both THC and CBD are metabolized by CYP3A4, meaning CYP3A4 inhibitors (antibiotics like clarithromycin/erythromycin, antifungals like itraconazole/ketoconazole, HIV medicines like ritonavir, and even grapefruit juice) can increase levels of THC, and CYP3A4 inducers (seizure medicines phenobarbital/phenytoin, the antibiotic rifampicin, St. John's Wort, and glucocorticoids like prednisone) can decrease levels of THC and CBD.

Thus, given all the potential interactions without clear evidence of actual interactions, how does one determine whether medical cannabis will interact with their own current medications? Essentially, based on available research, the likelihood of medical cannabis and CBD having significant interactions with medications (and vice versa) is very low, with a few exceptions. Patients on psychiatric medications, antibiotics, antifungals, antiseizure and HIV medicines should discuss this with their physician, but meaningful interactions are unlikely. However, there are a few medications where caution should be used with medical cannabis. *Warfarin* (Coumadin) is a blood thinner that interacts with many medications and needs to be monitored closely. CBD and THC can increase warfarin levels, and caution should be taken when using together. CBD increases the effects and the side effects of *clobazam*, a medication used for treating seizures in a rare disease called Lennox-Gastaut syndrome. CBD (Epidiolex) is also indicated for treating seizures in Lennox-Gastaut. When used together, levels of clobazam are increased, and thus side effects occur more frequently, so dosage may need to be lowered. *Valproate* is another drug used for seizures as well as migraines and bipolar disorder. However, when used with CBD, elevation of liver enzymes are observed, which can lead to liver injury.

Finally, while not an interaction, since medical cannabis can cause sleepiness, dizziness, and confusion, any medication or substance that also causes these symptoms can have additive effects. Alcohol, barbiturates, and benzodiazepines (alprazolam/Xanax) have these types of effects, so combinations of these substances with medical cannabis should be avoided or used with extreme caution. Interestingly, in a study of medical cannabis in patients using opioids (morphine and oxycodone), these additive effects were not seen, so use of cannabinoids and opioids simultaneously for treating pain is probably safe.

Chapter 11 Notes

1.   Active/Lethal Dose Ratio and Dependence Potential of Psychoactive Drugs. Data source: Gable, R. S. (2006). Acute toxicity of drugs versus regulatory status. In J. M. Fish (Ed.), *Drugs and Society: U.S. Public Policy*, 149–162, Lanham, MD: Rowman & Littlefield Publishers.

2.   National Academies of Sciences, Engineering, and Medicine. 2017. The Health Effects of Cannabis and Cannabinoids: The Current State of Evidence and Recommendations for Research. Washington, DC: The National Academies Press. https://doi.org/10.17226/24625.

3.   https://www.asam.org/resources/definition-of-addiction. Accessed 12/9/2019.

4.   Hasin, D. S., T. D. Saha, B. T. Kerridge, et al. Prevalence of Marijuana Use Disorders in the United States Between 2001-2002 and 2012-2013. *JAMA Psychiatry* 2015: 72(12), 1235–1242.

5.   Anthony, J. C., L. Warner, and R. Kessler. Comparative epidemiology of dependence on tobacco, alcohol, controlled substances and inhalants: basic findings from the National Comorbidity Survey. *Exp Clin Psychopharmacol* 1994: 2, 244–68.

6.   Russo, E. B., A. P. Mead, and D. Sulak. Current status and future of cannabis research. *Clinical Researcher* 2015: 29(2), 58–63.

7.   Ward, N. J., and L. Dye. "Cannabis and driving: a review of the literature and commentary." *Road Safety Research Report* 1999: 12.

8.   Lane, T., and W. Hall. Traffic fatalities within US states that have legalized recreational cannabis sales and their neighbours. *Addiction* 2019: 114(5), 847–856.

9.   Crume et al. Cannabis use during the perinatal period in a state with legalized recreational and medical marijuana: the association between maternal characteristics, breastfeeding patterns, and neonatal outcomes. *J Pediatr* 2018: 197, 90–96.

10.   Hickman et al. If cannabis caused schizophrenia—how many cannabis users may need to be prevented in order to prevent one case of schizophrenia? England and Wales calculations. *Addiction* 2009: 104, 1856–1861.

11. Kim, H. S., J. D. Anderson, O. Saghafi, K. J. Heard, A. A. Monte. Cyclic vomiting presentations following marijuana liberalization in Colorado. *Acad Emerg Med* 2015 Jun: 22(6), 694–9.

12. Whiting, P. F., et al. Cannabinoids for Medical Use: A Systematic Review and Meta-analysis. *JAMA* 2015: 313(24), 2456–2473.

13. Marinol package insert. https://www.accessdata.fda.gov/drugsatfda_docs/label/2017/018651s029lbl.pdf. Accessed 12/14/2019.

14. Sativex package insert. https://www.bayer.ca/omr/online/sativex-pm-en.pdf. Accessed 12/14/19.

15. Stout, S. M., and N. M. Cimino. Exogenous cannabinoids as substrates, inhibitors, and inducers of human drug metabolizing enzymes: a systematic review. *Drug metabolism reviews* 2014: 46(1), 86–95.

16. Epidiolex package insert. https://www.accessdata.fda.gov/drugsatfda_docs/label/2018/210365lbl.pdf. Accessed 12/14/2019.

17. Abrams, D. I., P. Couey, S. B. Shade, et al. Cannabinoid-opioid interaction in chronic pain. *Clin Pharmacol Ther.* 2011 Dec: 90(6), 844–51.

Part D:

Getting Medical Cannabis

Chapter 12:

Getting Medical Cannabis

In the previous sections of this book, we have discussed how medical cannabis and CBD work, some of the conditions they treat, the science and research behind medical cannabis and CBD, as well as how to use medical cannabis and CBD to treat medical conditions, especially in regard to strains, dosing, and titration to the desired effect. While this information should help patients use medical cannabis and CBD, one also needs to know how to legally obtain medical cannabis, which is not always a straightforward process and depends on the state you live in. This chapter will review how to obtain medical cannabis, which includes both registering with your state and getting certified by a clinician, as well as briefly describe the process for obtaining medical cannabis in a medical cannabis dispensary.

Legalization of Medical Marijuana

In order to understand some of the complexities of getting medical cannabis, it is important to understand how and where medical marijuana is legal. While marijuana was a legal component of tonics and elixirs in the United States in the early 1900s, the Controlled Substances Act of 1970 essentially made marijuana for medical use federally illegal, which remains the case today. Through the activism of HIV patients and caregivers in the 1990s, and with the passage of Proposition 215 in 1996, California became the first state where medical marijuana was legal. Over time, other states have also passed similar laws. Currently, medical marijuana is legal in thirty-three states and the District of Columbia.

In addition, there are many other states where medical marijuana is not broadly available but available with some restrictions. For example, Virginia recently passed laws allowing providers to certify patients, and growers and processors, to make products, though at the time of this writing, these processes are not currently in place. While marijuana, whether medicinal or recreational, is still illegal in the Commonwealth of Virginia, patients who are registered with Virginia's Board of Pharmacy who might be caught using marijuana will have "an affirmative defense," that essentially prevents them from being prosecuted. A list of the thirty-three states and DC and their associated medical cannabis websites is found at the end of this chapter.

In addition, eleven states (Alaska, California, Colorado, Illinois, Maine, Massachusetts, Michigan, Nevada, Oregon, Vermont, and Washington) and the District of Columbia have also legalized recreational marijuana. The politics and legality of recreational marijuana is beyond the scope of this book, which is written for patients who want to use medical cannabis to treat medical conditions. However, since recreational marijuana can be used medicinally, it is important to distinguish the difference in using marijuana in those eleven states and Washington, DC.

Medical cannabis is highly regulated by the state. That means that the quality, purity, and accuracy of the content are much more reliable than recreational marijuana. In states where both recreational and medical marijuana are legal, there are some advantages to medical cannabis over recreational marijuana: medical cannabis generally will cost less and have low to no taxes, there are usually higher limits to the amount of cannabis and/or THC that can be obtained, and qualified minors only have access to medical cannabis. One concerning development in states where medical cannabis was initially legal and recreational marijuana became subsequently legal relates to changes in the availability and costs of medical cannabis. While legalization of recreational marijuana may have decreased the cost of the marijuana plant (bud, flower), processed medical cannabis products like edibles and tinctures ending up becoming more expensive and less available.

Since the legality of medical cannabis is determined by the state, the rules in each state are slightly different. There are various boards that regulate medical cannabis; in some cases, this could be an existing board, or in other cases, an entirely new board is created. There are several areas that are regulated: regulations for those who grow the plant, regulations for those who process the plant into medicine, regulations for those who sell the plant (usually called dispensaries), regulations for clinicians who can certify patients, and finally regulations for patients, as well as their caregivers. The regulations surrounding each of these are complex, vary from state to state, and are beyond the scope of this book. However, while each state again is different, there are generally two things that patients need to do in every state in order to obtain medical cannabis: register with the state and get certified by a provider.

Registering with the State to Obtain Medical Cannabis

In almost every state, you need to register with that state and get certified by a medical provider. The order may or may not make a difference. In the District of Columbia, you must see a clinician first. In Maryland, the order doesn't matter, but both need to occur before medical cannabis can be obtained.

Registering with the state essentially means proving that you are a legal resident of that state. This will often mean having documents such as a driver's license or other forms to prove residence, such as a utility bill or property tax statement. More paperwork is often required if you do not have a driver's license for that state. Registration may be done by paper, online, both, or only one or the other. When done online, documents (like a picture of a driver's license or a passport photo) can be uploaded using a computer or cell phone. States also have provisions for caregivers. Caregivers are needed when a patient is not able to get medical cannabis by themselves because they are too frail, or if the patient is a minor, they will usually need an adult caregiver to obtain medical cannabis. The process for registering as a caregiver is usually similar to that of registering for the patient. There is often an extra step to ensure that a patient is linked to their caregiver. There is also usually some required payment in order to register. Payment is usually associated with obtaining a physical card, which often looks like a driver's license, that allows the patient or their caregiver to purchase and possess medical cannabis.

Getting Certified by a Medical Provider

In addition to registering with the state, you must be certified by a provider. Which type of provider can certify you, and the conditions that will qualify you for medical cannabis, also varies from state to state, but there is significant overlap. In general, the process for registering and the process for getting certified is often separate, with fees and renewal dates that are often distinct. For example, in Maryland, registration with the state (including a physical card) is $50 and lasts for three years. However, medical certification is required annually, and the fee varies based on what the certifying provider charges.

The job of the certifying provider is to ensure that the patient meets the criteria determined by the state that are acceptable to use medical cannabis. It is not the job of the certifying provider to diagnose a patient with a condition. Documentation of an established condition, such as a note from a doctor's visit or an x-ray report, is often required to establish that a patient has a given diagnosis. There are many qualifying conditions, which again vary by the state, but they often include diseases like cachexia (wasting), anorexia, severe or chronic pain, severe nausea, seizure disorders, muscle spasms, glaucoma, and post-traumatic stress disorder. Many patients have conditions that will respond to medical cannabis but don't meet the state's criteria. For this reason, most states have an "other" option. To qualify for a condition not listed by a state, the patient usually has to have medical condition that is severe, where other medical treatments have been ineffective, and the symptoms of the patient's conditions can be reasonably be expected to be relieved by the use of medical cannabis.

The types of providers that can certify patients also vary by state. While every state allows physicians to certify patients, most states allow some non-MD practitioners to certify such as nurses, dentists, physician assistants, nurse practitioners, and (in Washington, DC) naturopaths. Regardless of the type of clinician allowed to certify patients, the clinician must also be registered with the state to certify patients. The process for clinicians to register to certify patients also varies by state. In addition to proof of identify—for example, medical license number—some states require clinicians to complete training in medical cannabis before being able to certify patients.

Ideally, your regular health-care provider would be able to certify you for medical cannabis, but this is often not the case. Not only does your health-care provider have to register with your state to certify you, but she also has to be willing to do this. Unfortunately, not many health-care providers are willing to be certifying providers. There are a number of reasons that providers may not be willing to do this, including misunderstandings about the use of medical cannabis, relative lack of research compared to other more conventional methods, and liability concerns of recommending what is still a federally illegal substance. While Supreme Court precedent is pretty clear that clinicians who certify patients for medical cannabis in states where it is approved cannot have their licenses taken away, clinicians' ability to prescribe medications comes from the Drug Enforcement Agency (DEA), which is a federal institution. In fact, in the early years of medical cannabis legalization in Massachusetts, officers from DEA allegedly intimidated physicians who were certifying providers, showing up at their homes and offices, and threatened to take away their DEA licenses if they continued to certify patients for medical cannabis.[1]

Unfortunately, most certifying providers are usually separate from your regular doctor. They are often not physicians, usually only do medical cannabis certifications exclusively, and rarely take insurance. The other thing that is important to understand is that certifying providers are not usually required to give you specific recommendations of what cannabis products to take for your conditions, nor are they required to instruct you on proper use of specific products. Rather, certifying providers simply certify that you meet your state's criteria and provide you with the appropriate documentation that allows you access to the dispensary, where you can obtain medical cannabis. Finally, it is often difficult to find a certifying provider. Some state websites have lists, which are often not searchable by location or specialty. Thus, when choosing a certifying provider, I recommend the following steps. First, see if you regular doctor is able to certify, and if not, if he or she would be willing to do this for you. If this is not the case, I recommend finding a certifying physician who will not only give you the appropriate paperwork, but who is knowledgeable on the appropriate use of medical cannabis and can tell you exactly what to take for your condition (including knowing how cannabis interacts with the medications you are already on) and instruct you on exactly how to use medical cannabis. Unfortunately, there are very few physicians in many states who actually do this, which is one of the main reasons I decided to write this book.

Once you actually see a certifying provider, they will likely take a medical history and possibly perform a physical examination. They will likely have you fill out some paperwork, and will also likely ask to review some of your medical records, which document that you have the medical condition for which you are requesting medical cannabis use. The length of this process varies from provider to provider. Once the provider determines that you meet the state's criteria for medical cannabis, they will enter your name into the state's database and/or provide you with paperwork that enables you to get medical marijuana from a medical dispensary.

Medical Marijuana Dispensaries

Once you have finally registered with the state, have been certified by a medical provider, and have the proper documentation such as a card needed to obtain medical marijuana, you are now able to go into a medical marijuana dispensary. Medical marijuana dispensaries are regulated by the state in order to sell medical marijuana.

Going to a dispensary can be very overwhelming, especially for those who have never used recreational cannabis. There are often very many products to choose from. Since medical marijuana can be smoked (which I do not recommend), there is also often a significant amount of paraphernalia at dispensaries, which patients may be unaccustomed to seeing. Dispensaries can look very different, even in the same state. Some dispensaries are very "flower" focused, with jars of marijuana bud on display and chalkboards displaying which strains are on sale. Other dispensaries may be more medically focused and do not display any bud or flower, choosing to focus on products like edibles and tinctures. Some dispensaries can look very expensive, like a fancy clothing store, while others can look like a place to party. It's important that you choose a dispensary that you feel comfortable in and that can cater to your medical needs.

In many states, the dispensary will have two areas: a front area where any curious person can enter, and a back area or closed area, which only certified patients have access to. Because of the potential street value for stolen medical cannabis, security is usually very tight at a dispensary. It is not unusual to have armed personnel present or nearby, which again can be alarming to some patients. In both areas, the dispensary may have marketing materials, including vendors from various cannabis-related companies looking to sell patients on their various products.

In addition to the product itself, the main feature of the dispensary is the personnel that help you with the purchase. Like a pharmacist behind the counter, these dispensary employees are the ones who can help you pick the right product to use. Some dispensaries have special names for them, such as "patient care specialist." However, they are more commonly known as "budtenders." This nonclinical sounding name is likely derived from marijuana's recreational roots. The marijuana plant is commonly called "flower" or "bud," so the budtender "serves up" the bud, like a bartender at a bar or barista at a coffee shop. Budtenders can be quite important in the process of selecting the right product for you to use. Many are extremely knowledgeable and have been in the business for many years. Many budtenders in states where medical cannabis is only recently legal were imported from states like

California and Colorado, where medical cannabis has been used for a while. Since there is limited clinical data on which strains are best for which conditions, budtenders often have a level of knowledge that is not even found on the internet. Some of the recommendations I have used for patients (which is included in the last section of this book) have been developed not only based on a combination of clinical research and my experience with patients, but also from information I obtained from experienced and trustworthy budtenders.

As mentioned above, many, if not most, certifying providers do not give patients specific recommendations, but rather get patients the documentation needed to go to a dispensary, leaving the choice of product and instruction on its use to the budtender. However, while some budtenders have a great degree of expertise in the area of medical cannabis, there are several problems with using the budtender as the sole source of information in choosing medical cannabis products to treat specific conditions. First, there is no formal certification or degree for budtenders. Second, while some are extremely experienced and knowledgeable, you don't know if you are going to work with an experienced budtender or someone who just started working at the dispensary last week. Third, budtenders are not clinicians. They may be knowledgeable about different cannabis strains and conditions for which they might be effective. However, they don't have the clinical knowledge to know which products might work best in certain diseases, and they do not know which of your medications might interact with cannabis. Finally, medical cannabis is a business, and the budtender may have an inherent conflict in helping you choose the best product for you and generating revenue for the dispensary that pays their salary.

One of the main reasons that I wrote this book is because most certifying providers relegate clinical recommendations to the budtenders, which I do not think is wise. I started making handouts for my patients, which (in addition to specific recommendations that I hand out to each patient I certify) are designed to help them work with their budtender to pick out the most appropriate treatment for their specific conditions. These handouts turned into the last section of this book, in which I spell out specific recommendations to treat very common conditions that can be treated with medical cannabis. Thus, if you are able to get recommendations from your doctor about what to take for your condition, that is best. If not, you can use the information in the last section of this book and take it to your local budtender to help you choose the best products for you and your condition.

The Medical Cannabis Industry

Finding the right medical cannabis dispensary and choosing the right medical cannabis products can be confusing and overwhelming. However, it is important to understand that the medical cannabis industry is not just a bunch of mom-and-pop cannabis shops that grow and make their own products. While each state regulates growing, processing, and dispensing differently, the majority of medical cannabis dispensaries and products are owned and operated by a small list of large national companies. Given that more than half the states in the United States have legalized medical cannabis, and cannabis is entirely legal in Canada, investors see the cannabis and CBD market as a huge growth opportunity, and cannabis-related companies continue to merge to the point that medical cannabis, at least in the United States, is similar in many ways to most national businesses. Several large companies have cannabis farms, processing facilities, and dispensaries in multiple states. The main difference from other national companies (food, clothing) is that products sold in a given state must be grown and processed in the same state. The large companies essentially provide the infrastructure and back end to the local folks who own the licenses. Think of it like a McDonald's franchise, with the difference being that the meat for the burgers or the potatoes used to make the fries must come from the state where the restaurant is located. The fact that most cannabis dispensaries and products are limited to a small number of national vertically integrated companies is actually a good thing for patients, as it helps keep prices low and transparent, and keeps products consistent and of high quality. In addition, just like any brand of clothing (Levi's, for example) might have its own stores, but also may sell their products in other retail stores (e.g., Sears), products made by one company are not only sold in that company's dispensaries, but are also sold in other dispensaries owned by different companies. Finally, there are several online sites (Weedmaps, Leafly) where you can locate different products and dispensaries from any state and compare prices from product to product and dispensary to dispensary. Of course, you can only purchase medical cannabis products from dispensaries in the state where you are certified.

Additional Practical and Legal Issues

Since states regulate medical marijuana very differently, and all forms of marijuana are federally illegal, there are many complex practical and legal issues in regard to the use of medical cannabis. For example, due to banking regulations being under federal jurisdiction, most banks in the United States do not want to work with the dispensaries. For this reason, medical marijuana is a cash-only business. You usually cannot buy medical marijuana with a credit card, debit card, or check. For this reason, most dispensaries have an ATM machine at their locations.

There are also limits to how much cannabis one can purchase. The states will often determine how much cannabis a patient can purchase in a set period of time. For example, in the state of Maryland, a patient may purchase no more than 120 grams of dried flower (approximately four ounces) or 36 grams of THC in a thirty-day period.

There are laws about where you can use medical cannabis, even though it is legal in your state. You may be prohibited from using it in public. Since it is federally illegal, you can generally not use medical cannabis on federal property, such as a national park. If you live in an apartment or similar dwelling, you may have to abide by policies regarding medical cannabis use, even though it may be legal in your state. Also, employers are generally allowed to enforce rules (that you agree to before accepting employment) that may be different from the law. For example, if you are a police officer in a state where medical cannabis is legal, you still may not be allowed to use it, and you can even be tested for marijuana along with other drugs.

One of the complications about medical cannabis being federally illegal is that it cannot be taken across state lines. Medical cannabis is legal in both Maryland, where my main office is located, and the neighboring District of Columbia, where I also certify patients. However, it is technically illegal to take legally obtained medical cannabis from Maryland into DC, either by car or by foot. Probably the biggest issue involving travel is air travel. The airways and TSA are under federal jurisdiction. You cannot legally take medical cannabis onto an airplane, even if you are flying to a state where medical cannabis is legal. This is a huge challenge for patients who rely on medical cannabis to keep them well but must travel by plane. Another big issue for many is gun ownership. When you register to own a gun, you must attest that you do not use cannabis, and the required registration form is explicit that any form of marijuana cannot be used if trying to obtain a firearm.

A final concern is confidentiality. Every state requires that medical cannabis patients must register with that state, and this data is usually kept by the state on a secure server. In general, only those on the state's medical cannabis commission would have access to your data. It is highly unlikely that the federal government or any other authorities, such as the police, would ever have access to whether or not you are using medical cannabis. However, even if your private data is on a secure state government server, as there have been so many security breaches in so many sectors, almost no data is completely secure. Thus, if your privacy is extremely important to you, especially in regard to using cannabis, this is something you need to consider carefully before registering for using medical cannabis.

States Where Medical Marijuana Is Legal

Alaska
http://dhss.alaska.gov/dph/VitalStats/Pages/marijuana.aspx

Arizona
https://www.azdhs.gov/licensing/medical-marijuana/

Arkansas
https://www.healthy.arkansas.gov/

California
https://www.cdph.ca.gov/Programs/CHSI/Pages/MMICP.aspx

Colorado
https://www.colorado.gov/pacific/cdphe/medicalmarijuana

Connecticut
https://portal.ct.gov/DCP/Medical-Marijuana-Program/
Medical-Marijuana-Program

Delaware
https://dhss.delaware.gov/dph/hsp/medmarhome.html

Florida
https://knowthefactsmmj.com/

Hawaii
https://health.hawaii.gov/medicalcannabis/

Illinois
http://www.dph.illinois.gov/topics-services/prevention-wellness/
medical-cannabis

Louisiana
http://dhh.louisiana.gov

Maine
https://www.maine.gov/dafs/omp/medical-use/

Maryland
https://mmcc.maryland.gov/

Massachusetts
https://mass-cannabis-control.com/

Michigan
https://www.michigan.gov/lara/0,4601,7-154-79571_79575---,00.html

Minnesota
http://www.health.state.mn.us/topics/cannabis/

Missouri
https://health.mo.gov/safety/medical-marijuana/index.php

Montana
http://dphhs.mt.gov/qad/Licensure/MMP

Nevada
http://dpbh.nv.gov/Reg/Medical_Marijuana/

New Hampshire
http://www.dhhs.nh.gov/oos/tcp/index.htm

New Jersey
https://www.state.nj.us/health/medicalmarijuana/

New Mexico
https://nmhealth.org/about/mcp/svcs/

New York
https://www.health.ny.gov/regulations/medical_marijuana/

North Dakota
https://www.ndhealth.gov/mm/

Ohio
http://www.medicalmarijuana.ohio.gov/

Oklahoma
http://omma.ok.gov/apply-now

Oregon
https://www.oregon.gov/

Pennsylvania
https://www.pa.gov/guides/
pennsylvania-medical-marijuana-program/

Rhode Island
http://www.health.ri.gov/healthcare/medicalmarijuana/index.php

Utah
https://health.utah.gov/medical-cannabis

Vermont
https://medicalmarijuana.vermont.gov/

Washington
https://www.doh.wa.gov/YouandYourFamily/Marijuana/
MedicalMarijuana

Washington, DC

https://dchealth.dc.gov/service/
medical-marijuana-and-integrative-therapy

West Virginia

https://dhhr.wv.gov/bph/Pages/Medical-Cannabis-Program.aspx

Chapter 12 Notes

1. Lazar, K., and S. Murphy. "DEA targets doctors linked to medical marijuana." *The Boston Globe*, June 5, 2014. Accessed at https://www.bostonglobe.com/metro/2014/06/05/drug-enforcement-administration-targets-doctors-associated-with-medical-marijuana-dispensaries-physicians-say/PHsP0zRlaxXwnDazsohIOL/story.html on 4/21/2020.

Part E:

Treatment Recommendations for Specific Diseases and Conditions

Treatment Recommendations for Specific Diseases and Conditions
The following chapters are designed to give patients and their caregivers specific information about treating specific diseases. However, there are a few caveats to these recommendations, as well as some explanations regarding how these chapters were written that I believe are important to review before proceeding.

First, the recommendations are based on a combination of my own research, the results of patients whom I have treated, and conversations with other experts. These are general recommendations with substantial flexibility to account for different manifestations of a variety of clinical conditions. However, while I am a physician, I cannot give specific medical advice to specific individuals without reviewing their medical history or examining them. Thus, these recommendations should be considered as general advice only. I strongly recommend reviewing your treatment plan with your physician, even if your physician is not a certifying provider or lacks education regarding medical cannabis. In fact, you can share these recommendations with your provider to help choose which of these suggestions might work best for you, or which ones should be avoided, given your medical condition.

Second, these chapters are based on handouts that I give to my own patients that are meant to be stand-alone information that accompanies specific instructions I write down for them to take to the dispensary.

In addition, while I believe there is a wealth of information in the first sections of this book, I am also aware that many readers/patients will skip directly to these chapters. Thus, many of these chapters contain summaries of information previously discussed in this book. In other words, there is some purposeful redundancy in writing these chapters.

Third, while I have different recommendations for different conditions, and treat each individual patient with unique recommendations, there are some commonalities with many different clinical disorders as well as how medical cannabis may be helpful in these conditions. For example, insomnia can be a separate problem, or it can occur with either anxiety or depression. Thus, while there are separate chapters on insomnia, anxiety, and depression, you will find that some of the information in each of these chapters identical to the corresponding sections in these chapters regarding treating insomnia with medical cannabis.

Finally, there are so many conditions that can be improved using medical cannabis that it was impossible to write a chapter for every single one. The conditions I chose to write chapters about were based on the conditions I commonly see and treat with medical cannabis. For example, glaucoma is a condition known to be successfully treated with medical cannabis. However, I chose not to write a chapter on glaucoma primarily because I haven't treated many patients with glaucoma using cannabis. I believe the reason for this is that there are excellent prescription eye drops that are extremely effective for glaucoma and covered by insurance. Thus, I believe medical cannabis is likely only used for glaucoma in the rare instances that the eye drops aren't effective. The last two chapters are also meant to encompass a broader approach to cannabis use that can be applied to a variety of conditions—complex medical conditions like chronic fatigue and fibromyalgia, and use in the elderly, who generally have multiple medical conditions that occur simultaneously.

Chapter 13:

How to Use Medical Cannabis and CBD for Anxiety and PTSD

What Are Anxiety and PTSD?

Anxiety is more than just feeling worried. Patients commonly have associated symptoms such as changes in appetite and difficulty sleeping. In fact, anxiety disorders are the most common mental health conditions in the US, affecting forty million adults, or almost one-fifth of the population every year.[1] In addition, anxiety is not usually at a constant level. Patients may have more tolerable, lower levels of anxiety most days, but more severe episodes of panic more sporadically. Post-traumatic stress disorder, or PTSD, is different from anxiety in that it is usually occurs in patients that have experienced a traumatic event, and stimuli reminiscent of the traumatic event can trigger severe symptoms. While not everyone who experiences trauma will have PTSD, about eight million adults will have PTSD during a given year.[2] Patients with PTSD have flashbacks to the traumatic events, causing severe panic, and they can have nightmares that prevent them from sleeping soundly. PTSD is one of the qualifying conditions in most states that have legalized medical marijuana, and thus can respond very well to medical cannabis. However, while patients with general anxiety may be more likely to have daily symptoms and patients with PTSD are more likely to have more acute and severe symptoms, there can be significant overlap between the two, and treatment approaches can be similar. Thus, we will discuss both anxiety and PTSD in this chapter simultaneously.

Medical Cannabis for Anxiety and PTSD

Even though PTSD is a qualifying condition in many states, and anxiety is a very common problem for which many patients have found relief using medical cannabis, there is only limited data supporting the use Of medical cannabis for anxiety and PTSD . There are only limited clinical studies on the effects of cannabis on treating mood disorders. In studying medical cannabis, when THC was given to patients suffering from cancer, it was shown to have both an antianxiety effect as well as an antidepressant effects.[3] For patients with generalized anxiety disorder, nabilone, a synthetic version of THC not available in the United States, was studied and found to be more effective than placebo in reducing anxiety symptoms.[4] In addition, one study of eighty patients with PTSD, researchers found a 75% reduction in PTSD-related symptoms when using cannabis.[5] While more research is clearly needed, there is clearly a role for medical cannabis in the treatment of anxiety and PTSD. The endocannabinoid system regulates many functions of the body via multiple mechanisms, including interacting with the chemical messengers in the brain and nerves called neurotransmitters. The main neurotransmitters in the brain are serotonin, dopamine, and norepinephrine. Most prescription antianxiety medications work by modulating the effects of these neurotransmitters. We know that at least in animal studies, the cannabinoids in medical cannabis can have an effect on brain neurotransmitters as well.[6]

Strains for Anxiety and PTSD

While there are no randomized studies comparing the various strains of marijuana that have determined which is the most effective for anxiety or PTSD, patients who have anxiety generally prefer indica-based strains. While indica-based strains have both THC (the psychoactive component in marijuana that, at increased doses, can get patients "high") and CBD (the nonpsychoactive component), these strains are better at promoting relaxation and can also help with sleep, which is a common issue in patients with anxiety. In contrast, sativa strains can be stimulating, which is great for depression but may not be good for anxiety, and PTSD in particular. In addition, when picking a cannabis strain to help with anxiety, it is best to use a strain or product with terpenes that are relaxing and calming. Terpenes are some of the other substances in medical cannabis that, in addition to THC and CBD, can be a major determinant of their effect on the body. Beta-myrcene is an example of a terpene that can be used as a sedative and also has muscle-relaxing properties. Beta-myrcene can be found naturally in plants and herbs, and fruits such as mangoes. In addition to being sedative, myrcene has reported to have anti-inflammatory and analgesic properties. Limonene is another terpene that is excellent for patients with anxiety. Limonene is common in citrus fruits, and thus gives off a citrus scent. It can also be found in peppermint and rosemary, as well as cannabis. In addition to having antianxiety properties, limonene has a variety of effects on the body, including anticancer and antibacterial properties and may help with heartburn (gastroesophageal reflux). Finally, there are some terpenes that should be avoided. For example, alpha-Pinene can actually trigger anxiety. The following list includes several strains that patients with anxiety and PTSD have found effective:

Blue Dream and **OG Kush** are both sativa-predominant hybrid strains that have a medium (16–20%) amount of THC, with very little (<1%) CBD. Both contain myrcene as their predominant terpene, and OG Kush has some limonene. While sativa strains can be excellent for daytime use, since they can be stimulating, they should be used with caution in patients with severe anxiety, especially PTSD.

White Widow is a hybrid strain that has a medium amount of THC (14–18%) and very little (<1%) CBD. It works well for pain as well as anxiety. Its primary terpenes are the sedative myrcene, as well as caryophyllene, which is why it can also be used for pain.

ACDC is also a hybrid strain, which, like White Widow, is good for both pain and anxiety. However, it's known for having low levels of THC. It has the opposite ratio of White Widow, with a 20:1 CBD-to-THC ratio. Thus, this is one strain that should not make you "high."

Cannatonic is a balanced hybrid, but like ACDC, it has low (but slightly higher) amounts (3–7%) of THC, as well as medium amounts (6–10%) of CBD, with myrcene as a predominant terpene.

Granddaddy Purple (GDP) is a pure indica that has a medium (15–19%) amount of THC, with very little (<1%) CBD. GDP has myrcene and caryophyllene as terpenes and can be useful in both the anxiety and insomnia associated with depression.

Northern Lights is a pure indica strain with a medium (14–19%) amount of THC, and very little (<1%) CBD. Similar to GDP, it has myrcene and caryophyllene as its predominant terpenes, with a little bit of limonene. Northern Lights is also a relaxing, sleep-inducing strain that can simultaneously elevate mood. It is used for insomnia, pain relief, depression, and anxiety. It's also known for its mood-lifting effects.

CBD for Anxiety and PTSD

CBD is the nonpsychoactive cannabinoid in medical cannabis and is also found in hemp. While combinations of both THC and CBD can be effective for anxiety, CBD may be effective for anxiety and PTSD by itself. For general anxiety, the general feeling of being nervous or anxious is much more common than experiencing sudden bouts or severe anxiety or panic attacks. Physicians most commonly give pharmaceuticals to patients with depression and anxiety during the day that work by altering the levels of certain chemicals in the brain (such as serotonin and dopamine) that affect mood. These prescription medications can be effective but often have side effects. Some patients will report that while their anxiety or depression is improved, they have a "brain fog" or simply don't feel like themselves. CBD can help relieve symptoms of anxiety, but without the side effects of medications. While there are a few small studies that show high-dose CBD might reduce acute anxiety before a stressful event, such as public speaking,[7] CBD has better evidence if taken on a daily basis, at lower doses (around 25 mg daily) to reduce general anxiety.[8] PTSD is related to anxiety, and in one small study, there was significant improvement in symptoms when patients with PTSD took daily CBD.[9]

While you can either use cannabis-derived CBD or hemp-derived CBD for daily treatment of anxiety, I generally recommend hemp-derived CBD because it is usually less expensive, and you can obtain this without certification. However, because hemp-derived CBD is not regulated by the FDA, you must be very careful that you are getting a high-quality, full-spectrum, third-party verified product. For the treatment of anxiety, I recommend 25 to 30 mg of CBD a day, which can be obtained by using CBD oil/tincture under the tongue, or CBD oil capsules. CBD, in general, does not immediately alleviate anxiety or PTSD, but rather, taken daily for at least one to two weeks, it can start to affect some of the chemical signaling in the brain to help alleviate symptoms. Thus, don't expect to see improvement in symptoms right away.

Using Different Formulations for Anxiety and PTSD

Almost as important as which strain of cannabis you use, or other factors such as the ratio of THC to CBD, the formulation you use to treat anxiety is also very important. This is because different formulations have different onsets of actions and different durations. Patients with severe and acute anxiety, especially with panic attacks and PTSD, will need something that works very quickly. However, patients with general anxiety can have symptoms that are present all day; thus, a longer-lasting agent will be needed.

Pills or capsules (edibles) take longer to work (about an hour), but last longer in the body (up to eight hours). Thus, edibles are not very effective for acute anxiety symptoms, but for patients who have daily anxiety symptoms, edibles can be particularly helpful. Edibles may also be needed for patients with anxiety or PTSD who have difficulty staying asleep. Depending on the state, some edibles may be available as an indica, sativa, or hybrid, and may even be available in a specific strain.

Vape comes in the form of a concentrated liquid (called "**concentrate**") that is extracted from the cannabis plant, and usually heated so it can be inhaled. Thus, vape is a way to inhale cannabis without smoking it. Vape also works very quickly (seconds to minutes), which is very beneficial for patients who have acute anxiety or panic. Another advantage of vape is that you can also get the full extract of a particular cannabis plant strain, gaining the benefit of all the cannabinoids and terpenes from the plant without smoking. Almost all cannabis strains are available in vape or concentrate, and you can choose one of those listed above (or similar) to start with. However, vape doesn't last very long (an hour or so), meaning that patients who have anxiety symptoms throughout the day will likely also need something that is longer lasting.

Tinctures are liquids that come in droppers. You drop tincture under your tongue to allow for faster absorption than swallowing them directly. Tinctures take about thirty minutes to work, and last four to six hours. Thus, tinctures can be a good option for people who have both acute anxiety and anxiety throughout the day, especially if they would like to use one product for both issues. Tinctures are also slightly easier to titrate (adjust the dose), as they can be increased drop by drop. Finally, while this varies state by state, while most tinctures are extractions of primarily THC and CBD, some tinctures are available in sativa, indica, or hybrid strains, and some states sell extracts of the whole cannabis plant, so you can use a specific strain, like the ones listed above.

General Recommendations for Treating Anxiety and PTSD

In considering the treatment of anxiety with medical cannabis, it is best to divide symptoms into three categories: daytime anxiety, difficulty sleeping at night, and acute or sudden episodes of panic. All of these can be seen in patients with both general anxiety and PTSD, though not every patient will experience all three. In addition, it is not uncommon for individual patients with anxiety or PTSD to have one of these areas that is more severe. Thus, in treating patients, it is often best to start by first focusing on that particular area. However, when there are multiple areas of difficulty, in general, focusing on sleep is the best place to start, as once sleep is improved, especially in patients with PTSD bothered by nightmares, anxiety naturally starts to improve.

1. **Treat general anxiety and PTSD by taking a high-dose CBD capsule pill or tincture every day.**

   Because there is good evidence that CBD alone can help with anxiety, I recommend that every patient with anxiety or PTSD take daily CBD. Start with 25 to 30 mg of CBD a day in a pill/edible/capsule or tincture. This can either be a cannabis-derived CBD or pure-hemp-derived CBD. I generally recommend hemp-derived CBD, as it is less expensive, easier to obtain, and because there is virtually no THC, it will not make you sleepy or high.

2. **Address sleep issues by using nighttime cannabis with higher doses of THC, ideally with CBN.**

   Insomnia is a common symptom of anxiety and especially PTSD, and a lack of a good night's sleep can contribute to further symptoms. Fortunately, cannabis is also very good at making people sleepy. In addition, to THC and CBD, there is also CBN, which stands for cannabinol. Like CBD, CBN is a nonpsychoactive cannabinoid, and CBN is particularly good for sleep. Five milligrams of CBN may be as effective as a 10 mg dose of diazepam (generic for Valium) for inducing sleep. There are several edibles and tinctures sold throughout the country that are available in a 1:1 ratio of CBN:THC. Some of these also contain terpenes and other natural components, such as organic chamomile or melatonin, that when combined with THC and CBN, can be quite effective to help induce sleep. Since tinctures only take about twenty to thirty minutes to work, and last about four to six hours, a 1:1 CBN:THC tincture is often a great place to start, as it can help you fall asleep and stay asleep. Check the milligrams per milliliter on the bottle to ensure you are getting the correct amount. For example, a 15 ml bottle with 50 mg of THC has over 3mg THC per dropperful, so start with ½ dropperful 30 minutes before bedtime, and increase by a ¼ to ½ dropperful each evening until you are falling asleep easily and staying asleep.

For patients who fall asleep just fine but get up early in the morning and can't fall back asleep ("terminal insomnia"), or patients with PTSD who are suddenly awakened by nightmares, a pill or edible may be a better option. While pills or edibles take about an hour to start working, they last for six to eight hours. Start with an edible that contains 5 mg of THC, ideally from an indica strain. Some edibles will also contain components like melatonin to aid with sleep. Start with a half tablet for the first night or two. If that does not work, then increase the dose to a full tablet before bedtime. You can increase by half a tablet every two nights until you are staying asleep through the night.

For patients who have racing thoughts once they get in bed and turn off the lights, a vape or concentrate can also be used, since it works immediately. Indica strains like GDP usually work best. Start with one puff a few minutes before bedtime. You can increase by a puff every few minutes until you feel yourself getting sleepy. Patients who have problems both falling asleep and staying asleep (terminal insomnia, nightmares) can use both a vape right before bed to help them fall asleep, as well as an edible right before bedtime to keep them asleep. Finally, when using medical cannabis to help you sleep, do not forget about good sleeping habits (known as sleep hygiene): turn off the lights, do not watch TV in bed, and do not consume caffeine after 4:00 p.m.

3. **Use an indica or hybrid concentrate/vape for acute anxiety symptoms.**

Vape (also known as concentrate) is likely the best option for acute episodes of anxiety. A hybrid strain like ACDC or Cannatonic that is low in THC may be particularly effective for daytime anxiety. An indica strain like Granddaddy Purple has more THC and thus is stronger and more relaxing but can also be sedating. When symptoms of anxiety occur, start with one puff, and wait a few minutes to see how the cannabis affects you. You can slowly increase by one puff at a time. Eventually, you will figure out the number of puffs it takes to relax you without making you sleepy or "high."

4. **For patients that have constant, daily anxiety, use hybrid edibles or tinctures two to three times a day.**

   For many patients that I treat with anxiety, the combination of daily CBD, vape for acute symptoms, and medical cannabis to address sleep issues is all that is needed to successfully treat anxiety and PTSD. However, some patients have anxiety throughout the day, and despite using medical cannabis as above, they have persistent daily symptoms. Those patients can add edibles or tinctures two to three times a day to control these persistent symptoms. While edibles and tinctures come in a variety of ratios of CBD to THC (14:1, 4:1, 1:1, 1:4, et cetera), since I recommend that patients take higher doses of daily CBD, I have found it much easier (and less expensive) for patients to stick with 2.1 or 1:1 products. Since pills and tinctures are often reconstituted with terpenes added back, chose products specifically designed for anxiety, which have terpenes such as beta-myrcene and limonene. While each state is different, some companies make edibles and tinctures that are either sativa, indica, or hybrid. Though indicas tend to be better for anxiety (and sativas can actually make anxiety worse), indicas are also sedating. Thus, I recommend using a low-dose hybrid edible or tincture if using throughout the day. In addition, some companies in some states even make strain-specific products, so you can use one of the hybrid strains listed above (White Widow, ACDC, Cannatonic). Start with approximately 0.5 to 1 mg of THC for the first dose. You can figure out how much THC is in one pill or one dropperful of tincture by looking at the package. For example, a 2:1 tincture that comes in a 15 ml bottle with 300 mg cannabinoids, half a dropperful (0.5 ml, or 10 drops) contains 10 mg of cannabinoids.

So 3 drops will be about 2 mg of CBD and 1 mg THC. You can start with about 5 drops (1–2 mg of THC) each day, or even with each dose, and then slowly increase the amount of THC drop by drop until you get the desired amount of anxiety relief without side effects. Edibles are easier to dose because the milligrams are stated on the package, and you can usually easily cut an edible in half or quarter to achieve your desired dose. Most patients achieve good results at 2 to 15 mg of THC per dose.

5. **Use nonmedicinal approaches in addition to cannabinoids.**
   While beyond the scope of a book like this, it is worth mentioning that in addition to medicinal treatments for anxiety (including pharmaceuticals like Prozac or Xanax, or natural products like medical cannabis), nonmedicinal treatments are also very effective. Meditation, yoga, and exercise are all examples of nonmedicinal treatments for anxiety. In addition, therapy with a trained professional (psychiatrist, psychologist, or counselor) is often very effective. Studies that have compared medicines to therapy usually find them equally effective, and in fact, find the combination of both therapy and medication to be the most effective option.

6. **Don't stop daily prescription medications right away.**
   Many patients I see with anxiety (as well as depression) are already taking prescription medications. While it might be wonderful if patients can treat their medical conditions without prescriptions, I believe the goal should be to first improve symptoms. I recommend that patients generally stay on their medications when starting with medical cannabis until they are feeling better. While certain medicines that are supposed to be taken as needed, like benzodiazepines (Xanax/alprazolam, Valium/diazepam) and sedatives for sleep (Ambien/zolpidem), can be quickly replaced by cannabis, other medications meant to be taken daily, like SSRIs (Prozac/fluoxetine, Zoloft/sertraline, Lexapro/escitalopram) and bupropion (Wellbutrin) should not be stopped. Stopping these

medicines immediately can make patients very sick. If you are using medical cannabis and CBD successfully, and are interested in trying to get off your daily prescription medication, please speak with your doctor first before doing so.

Chapter 13 Notes

1. Anxiety and Depression Association of America (ADAA): Facts & Statistics. https://adaa.org/about-adaa/press-room/facts-statistics. Accessed 5/25/2020.

2. PTSD: National Center for PTSD. https://www.ptsd.va.gov/ understand/common/common_adults.asp. Accessed 5/25/2020.

3. Regelson, W., J. R. Butler, J. Schulz, T. Kirk, L. Peek, M. L. Green, and M. O. Zalis. Delta 9-THC as an effective antidepressant and appetite-stimulating agent in advanced cancer patients. In M. C. Braude and S. Szara (Eds.), *The Pharmacology of Marihuana* (pp. 763–776). New York: Raven Press, 1976.

4. Fabre, L. F., and D. McLendon. The efficacy and safety of nabilone (a synthetic cannabinoid) in the treatment of anxiety. *J Clin Pharmacol* 1981 Aug–Sep: 21(S1), 377S–382S.

5. Greer, G. R., C. S. Grob, and A. L. Halberstadt. PTSD symptom reports of patients evaluated for the New Mexico Medical Cannabis Program. *J Psychoactive Drugs* 2014 Jan–Mar: 46(1), 73–7.

6. Banerjee, S. P., S.H. Snyder, and R. Mechoulam. Cannabinoids: influence on neurotransmitter uptake in rat brain synaptosomes. *J Pharmacol Exper Therap* 1975: 194, 74–81.

7. Bergamaschi, M. M., R. H. Queiroz, et al. Cannabidiol reduces the anxiety induced by simulated public speaking in treatment-naïve social phobia patients. *Neuropsychopharmacology* 2011 May: 36(6), 1219–26.

8. Shannon, S., et al. Cannabidiol in Anxiety and Sleep: A Large Case Series. *Perm J* 2019: 23, 18–41.

9. Elms, L., S. Shannon, S. Hughes, and N. Lewis. Cannabidiol in the Treatment of Post-Traumatic Stress Disorder: A Case Series. *Journal of Alternative & Complementary Medicine* 2019 Apr: 25(4), 392–397.

Chapter 14:

How to Use Medical Cannabis and CBD for Insomnia

Insomnia Is a Common Problem

Insomnia is a common problem for many adults and children. About fifty to seventy million Americans are affected by chronic sleep disorders and intermittent sleep problems that can significantly diminish health, alertness, and safety.[1] There are many prescription products (Ambien/zolpidem) and supplements (melatonin) that are successful in many patients. However, for some, these treatments either do not work or have unwanted side effects. In the case of Ambien (zolpidem is the generic name), while generally safe, there are rare instances that have occurred where patients who have used this medication have gotten out of bed and driven vehicles, prepared and eaten food, made phone calls, and even had sexual encounters while not fully awake. These patients usually do not even remember these events. Fortunately, medical cannabis can help with insomnia and is not associated with these types of side effects.

Types of Insomnia

Patients with insomnia can either have problems falling asleep, staying asleep, or both. When it comes to staying asleep, one type of insomnia that is commonly associated with depression occurs when patients wake up early in the morning (e.g., 4:00 a.m.) and have problems falling back to sleep. This is often known as "terminal insomnia." It is not called "terminal" because it is life threatening, but rather because the insomnia comes at the end, or "termination," of the sleep cycle. In contrast, problems falling asleep are usually more associated with anxiety. The patients are generally very tired at the end of the day, but once they attempt to go to sleep, they have racing thoughts or worries, which prevent them from sleeping. Also, it is not uncommon for patients to have problems both falling asleep and staying asleep. Finally, there are other contributing factors to insomnia. In addition to habits that do not promote sleep, such as taking medications or eating foods that can keep you awake, there are medical conditions such as restless leg syndrome and pain that can keep people awake. Different types of medical cannabis, particularly regarding formulations, should be used for different types of sleeping problems.

Medical Cannabis for Insomnia

While there is surprisingly limited research on medical cannabis and sleep, sedation is very much a known effect of THC. Thus, it is not surprising that many patients using medical cannabis do so, at least in part, for the purposes of assistance with sleep. One interesting finding that confirms this is an analysis in Colorado, a state where both medical cannabis and recreational marijuana have been legal for several years, which showed that sales of over-the-counter medications for sleep decreased shortly after the opening of recreational marijuana dispensaries.[2] A study in rats showed that vaporized cannabis improved sleep, but only in the early phase.[3] In regard to human studies, an Israeli study of 128 adults fifty years of age and older found that the use of medical cannabis was associated with improvements in sleeping through the night.[4] This highlights an importance in the use of medical cannabis for insomnia, which is that formulation (e.g., inhaled versus edible) likely matters, as faster-acting agents are better for assistance in falling asleep, whereas longer-acting agents are needed to maintain sleep in patients with terminal insomnia.

Strains for Insomnia

While there are no randomized studies comparing the various strains of marijuana that have determined which is the most effective for insomnia, patients who have insomnia generally prefer indica-based strains. While indica-based strains have both THC (the psychoactive component in marijuana that, at increased doses, can get patients "high") and CBD (the nonpsychoactive component), these strains are better at promoting relaxation and sleep. In addition, when picking a cannabis strain to help one sleep, it is best to use a strain or product with terpenes that help promote sleep. Terpenes are some of the other substances in medical cannabis that, in addition to THC and CBD, can be a major determinant of their effect on the body. Beta-myrcene is an example of a terpene that can be used as a sedative and muscle relaxant. Beta-myrcene can be found naturally in plants and herbs, and fruits such as mangoes. In addition to being sedative, myrcene has reported to have anti-inflammatory and analgesic properties.

Blue Cheese is an indica-predominant (80%) hybrid strain. It also has a medium (14–18%) amount of THC, and very little (<1%) CBD. While it has caryophyllene and some myrcene like GDP and Northern Lights, its primary terpene is limonene. This, as well as the small sativa component, gives it a tiny bit of uplifting feeling, and thus can be used in insomnia associated with anxiety and depression. The following are two strains that patients with insomnia have found particularly effective:

Granddaddy Purple (GDP) is a pure indica that has a medium (15–19%) amount of THC, with very little (<1%) CBD. GDP has myrcene and caryophyllene as terpenes, and can be useful in both the anxiety and insomnia associated with depression.

Northern Lights is a pure indica strain with a medium (14–19%) amount of THC, and very little (<1%) CBD. Similar to GDP, it has myrcene and caryophyllene as its predominant terpenes, with a little bit of limonene. Northern Lights is also a relaxing, sleep-inducing strain that can simultaneously elevate mood. It is used for insomnia, pain relief, depression, and anxiety. It's also known for its mood-lifting effects.

CBD for Insomnia

CBD is the nonpsychoactive cannabinoid in medical cannabis and is also found in hemp. It is known to be effective for anxiety,[5] which is common for people who have insomnia. However, using CBD as a sleep aid is questionable. CBD is usually taken as a tincture (liquid) or pill (liquid capsule) form and in general does not work immediately, but rather, when taken daily, shows effects in about one to two weeks. However, I have several patients that tell me when taking CBD, especially as a tincture, before bedtime, they find it relaxing, which subsequently helps them fall sleep. When it comes to depression and anxiety, CBD appears to work by modifying the brain's neurotransmitters, in the same way prescriptions work. One of the benefits to prescription treatments for anxiety and depression is that they improve sleep. Thus, for patients who primarily have insomnia, but may have a component of anxiety or depression, daily CBD might help. While you can either use marijuana-derived CBD or hemp-derived CBD for daily treatment, I generally recommend hemp-derived CBD because it is usually less expensive, and you can obtain this without certification. However, because hemp-derived CBD is not regulated by the FDA, you must be very careful that you are getting a high-quality, full-spectrum, third-party-verified product. For insomnia that is associated with either anxiety or depression, I recommend 25 to 30 mg of CBD each evening, preferably used in tincture form, taken under the tongue, as this may increase onset of action.

Using Different Formulations for Insomnia

Almost as important as which strain of cannabis you use, or other factors such as the ratio of THC to CBD, the formulation you use to treat insomnia is also important. This is because different formulations have different onsets of actions and different durations. Patients with insomnia who have problems falling asleep need something that works quickly, whereas patients who have problems staying asleep need something that has a longer duration.

Pills or capsules (edibles) take longer to work (about an hour hour), but last longer in the body (up to eight hours), so some type of edible is usually needed for patients who have difficulty staying asleep. Depending on the state, some edibles may be available as an indica, sativa, or hybrid and may even be available in a specific strain.

Vape comes in the form of a concentrated liquid (called "**concentrate**") that is extracted from the marijuana plant, and usually heated so it can be inhaled. Thus, vape is a way to inhale cannabis without smoking it. Vape also works very quickly (seconds to minutes), which is very beneficial for patients who have difficulty falling asleep. Another advantage of vape is that you can also get the full extract of a particular cannabis plant strain, gaining the benefit of all the cannabinoids and terpenes from the plant, without smoking. Almost all cannabis strains are available in vape or concentrate, and you can choose one of those listed above (or similar) to start with. However, vape doesn't last very long (an hour or so), meaning that patients who have problems staying asleep as well as falling asleep will need something in addition to vape to treat both types of insomnia.

Tinctures are liquids that come in droppers. You drop a tincture under your tongue to allow for fast absorption rather than swallowing them directly. Tinctures take about thirty minutes to work, and last four to six hours. Thus, tinctures can be a good option for people who have issues both falling asleep and staying asleep, and who would like to use one product for both issues. Tinctures are also slightly easier to titrate (adjust the dose), as they can be increased drop by drop. Finally, while this varies state by state, while most tinctures are extractions of primarily THC and CBD, some tinctures are available in sativa, indica, or hybrid strains, and some states sell extracts of the whole cannabis plant, so you can use a specific strain, like the ones listed above.

General Recommendations for Insomnia

1. **Use medical cannabis vape (or tincture) to help you fall asleep.**

Both vape (concentrate) or tinctures (see below) can help with falling asleep, but for those who primarily have issues primarily falling asleep, vape is probably best. Since it works immediately, vape can help patients who have racing thoughts once they get in bed and turn off the lights. In addition, some patients with problems falling asleep, possibly due to stress or anxiety, simply have problems "winding down," even before attempting to go to sleep, which vape can be helpful for, even in the late afternoon or early evening. Indica strains, like the ones listed above, generally work best. Start with one puff a few minutes before bedtime. You can increase by a puff every few minutes until you feel yourself getting sleepy.

2. **Use a medical cannabis edible (or tincture) to help you stay asleep.**
   Fortunately, cannabis is very good at making people sleepy. In addition to THC and CBD, there is also CBN, which stands for cannabinol. Like CBD, CBN is a nonpsychoactive cannabinoid, and CBN is particularly good for sleep. Five milligrams of CBN may be as effective as a 10-mg dose of diazepam (generic for Valium) for inducing sleep. There are several edibles and tinctures throughout the country that are available in a 1:1 ratio of CBN:THC. Some of these also contain terpenes and other natural components, such as organic chamomile or melatonin, that when combined with THC and CBN, can be quite effective to help induce sleep. For patients who fall asleep just fine but get up early in the morning and can't fall back asleep ("terminal insomnia"), a pill or edible may be a better option. While pills or edibles take about an hour to start working, they last for six to eight hours. Start with an edible that contains 5 mg of THC, ideally from an indica strain and/or one that has a 1:1 CBN:THC ratio. As mentioned, some edibles will also contain components like melatonin to aid with sleep. Start with a half tablet for the first night or two. If that does not work, then increase the dose to a full tablet before bedtime. You can increase by half a tablet every two nights until you are staying asleep through the night.

3. **Use a medical cannabis tincture for problems both falling and staying asleep, or consider vape plus an edible for more severe combined insomnia.**

Since tinctures only take about twenty to thirty minutes to work, and last about four to six hours, a 1:1 CBN:THC tincture is often a great place to start for patients with insomnia, as it can help you fall asleep and stay asleep. Check the milligrams per milliliter on the bottle to ensure you are getting the correct amount. For example, a 15 ml bottle with 50 mg of THC has over 3 mg of THC per dropperful, so start with ½ a dropperful 30 minutes before bedtime, and increase by a ¼ to ½ dropperful each evening until you are falling asleep easily and staying asleep.

However, if tinctures don't work, or if your insomnia is so severe you need something that works right away to help you fall asleep, you may want to consider a combination of both a vape to help you fall asleep and an edible to help you stay asleep. Since the edible is being used for staying asleep, you can take both the vape and edible right before bedtime. The vape will get you to fall asleep pretty quickly and should last for about an hour. Around the hour mark, the edible should start working to keep you asleep. In general, when using medical cannabis, I advise patients to start low and go slow. If you decide to start with both a vape and an edible simultaneously, this is doubly true, especially with the edible. Titrate, or slowly increase, the doses of both to get the desired effect as described above, but perhaps start even lower with the edible (e.g., one-fourth of a pill the first night).

4. **Consider daily CBD, especially if anxiety may be a component of your insomnia.**

As mentioned, CBD is the component of cannabis that is not sedating. It is not supposed to make you sleepy. However, anxiety and insomnia are often connected, and since CBD can be very effective in treating anxiety, a trial of CBD in addition to the above recommendations, and especially if the above recommendations aren't working, should be considered. For insomnia that is associated with either anxiety or depression, I recommend 25 to 30 mg of full-spectrum hemp-based CBD each evening, preferably used in tincture form, taken under the tongue, as this may increase onset of action.

5. Address other factors that may be contributing to the insomnia.

One significant contributor to insomnia is poor sleep habits (also known as sleep hygiene). It is important to have good sleep hygiene, especially if you have insomnia. This includes turning out the lights before getting into bed and turning the TV off before getting into bed. In fact, those with insomnia shouldn't even watch the TV or read in bed. The body needs to "learn" that the bed should only be used for sleep. Certain foods, especially caffeine, can keep people awake at night. If caffeine can't be avoided, it shouldn't be used after 4:00 p.m. Some patients use alcohol to help them sleep. While a glass of wine with dinner can be enjoyable and even have some health benefits, alcohol should not be used as a sleep inducer. Cannabis is actually safer and more effective. It is important to note that using alcohol with cannabis can cause disequilibrium (the "spins"), which can be quite unsettling. Finally, some patients have restless leg syndrome, in which their legs simply cannot stop moving when trying to go to sleep. In addition to using marijuana products at bedtime that have terpenes that relax muscles, sometimes topical cannabis formulations can help with leg movements.

Chapter 14 Notes

1. https://www.sleepfoundation.org/articles/sleep-studies. Accessed 5/25/2020.

2. Doremus, J. M., S. S. Stith, and J. M. Vigil. Using recreational cannabis to treat insomnia: Evidence from over-the-counter sleep aid sales in Colorado. *Complement Ther Med* 2019: 47, 102207.

3. Mondino, A., M. Cavelli, J. Gonzalez, et al. Acute effect of vaporized Cannabis on sleep and electrocortical activity. *Pharmacol Biochem Behav* 2019: 179, 113–123.

4. Sznitman, S. R., S. Vulfsons, D. Meiri, and G. Weinstein. Medical cannabis and insomnia in older adults with chronic pain: a cross-sectional study. *BMJ support. palliat. care* 2020.

5. Shannon, S., et al. Cannabidiol in Anxiety and Sleep: A Large Case Series. *Perm J* 2019: 23, 18–041.

Chapter 15:

How to Use Medical Cannabis and CBD for Depression

Depression Is a Common Problem

Depression is extremely common in the United States, with over 10% of adults having it over the course of a lifetime.[1] It is more common in women than men, and there is a genetic component as well. Most patients with depression are not seen by a psychiatrist, but rather will be diagnosed by their primary care physician.[2] Depression is often triggered by a stressful life event, though that is not always the case. In addition to genetics, there are other factors that put patients at risk, such as being socially isolated. Symptoms of depression include depressed mood, loss of interest or pleasure, change in appetite or weight, sleep abnormalities, fatigue, and problems concentrating.

Insomnia Is Common with Depression

One of the most common symptoms associated with depression is insomnia.[3] Patients with depression can either have problems falling asleep, staying asleep, or both. However, a common form of insomnia associated with depression occurs when patients wake up early in the morning (e.g., 4:00 a.m.) and have problems falling back to sleep. This is often known as "terminal insomnia." It is not called "terminal" because it is life threatening, but rather because the insomnia comes at the end, or "termination," of the sleep cycle.

Sleep issues, and terminal insomnia in particular, can lead to sleepiness or sluggishness during the day, which can make symptoms of depression even worse.

Anxiety Is Common with Depression

While anxiety and depression are considered two separate entities, these medical illnesses often occur together. Patients with anxiety can have similar symptoms to depression (insomnia, depressed mood), and patients with depression can have periods of anxiousness. The overlap of both conditions and symptoms likely stem from a similar cause to both conditions. Patients with both anxiety and depression often have a family history of mental illness, so there is usually a genetic component that predisposes patients.[4] Often triggered by a stressful event or events, changes in brain chemistry affect a patient's mood, leading to depression, anxiety, or both. Pharmaceutical treatments have been targeted at reversing these changes in neurotransmitters—the biochemicals in our brains that help with mood and thought—which include dopamine, serotonin, and norepinephrine. CBD and THC work on similar pathways in the brain that medications used to treat depression do, and they can also improve changes in neurotransmitters, though without the side effects that can occur with prescription drugs.

Medical Cannabis for the Treatment of Depression

While there is evidence for the role of medical cannabis in anxiety and insomnia, which are both associated with depression, and neurotransmitters, which can be affected by cannabis, are involved in all three entities, the research regarding medical cannabis for the treatment of the depression is less robust. In one study of patients suffering from cancer, when THC was given to these patients, it was shown to have both an antianxiety effect as well as antidepressant effects.[6] In studying medical cannabis for use specifically for depression, the evidence is both limited and shows mixed results.[7] There is slightly more evidence to support the use of CBD in depression. However, research on both animals and humans indicates that CBD may have antidepressant properties as well.[8, 9] Nonetheless, given its role in affecting neurotransmitters, its efficacy in treating both anxiety and insomnia, and limited research in humans and animals that it can be effective, medical cannabis is a viable option for patients suffering from depression, especially when pharmaceutical and behavioral treatments are not working.

Strains for Depression

Marijuana contains many different substances (called cannabinoids) that have medicinal properties. In addition to THC (the component that can make you "high") and CBD (which does not make you high), there are substances called terpenes that give marijuana its smell and flavor. The combination and proportion of cannabinoids and terpenes will help determine which strains are best to treat your depression. The most common way of classifying strains is indica and sativa. Sativa strains are generally uplifting and energizing, while indica strains are generally more relaxing and sedating. Thus, it is not surprising that some of the sativa strains tend to be better for patients with depression. There are also hybrid strains, which can be balanced (half indica/half sativa) or more predominant in one. There are several sativa-predominant hybrids, which are useful in depression, and because they are energizing, they are also popular for daytime use. Indicas can be useful for the insomnia and anxiety components of depression. While there are many terpenes that are helpful for depression, limonene and myrcene can be particularly useful. Limonene is also found in citrus fruits and may be beneficial for depression, anxiety, pain, and inflammation. Myrcene is another terpene, which can also be found in hops, mango, and lemongrass and can cause relaxation. While the various strains and terpenes can be effective for depression, every patient is different, so it may take some trial and error to determine which strain is the right strain for you. Below are a few strains that patients have successfully used for depression.

Jack Herer and **Green Crack** are both sativa strains that have a medium (15–19%) amount of THC, with very little (<1%) CBD. Both contain the terpene caryophyllene, which is useful in neve pain as well as depression.

Blue Dream and **OG Kush** are both sativa-predominant hybrid strains that have a medium (16–20%) amount of THC, with very little (<1%) CBD. Both contain myrcene, and OG Kush has some limonene.

Harlequin is also a sativa-dominant hybrid, but with a much higher CBD-to-THC ratio (about 5:2). It has low amounts (3–6%) of THC, and medium amounts (7–10%) of CBD. Harlequin is high in myrcene as well, and along with Green Crack, it is helpful for chronic fatigue.

Cannatonic is a balanced hybrid, but like Harlequin, it has low amounts (3–7%) of THC, and medium amounts (6–10%) of CBD, with myrcene as a predominant terpene.

Granddaddy Purple (GDP) is a pure indica that has a medium (15–19%) amount of THC, with very little (<1%) CBD. GDP has myrcene and caryophyllene as terpenes, and can be useful in both the anxiety and insomnia associated with depression.

CBD for Depression

CBD is the nonpsychoactive cannabinoid in medical cannabis and is also found in hemp. It is known to be effective for anxiety,[10] which is a common with depression. However, while CBD's effects on depression are less well known, animal and human research suggest that it may be helpful.[9] While you can either use marijuana-derived CBD or hemp-derived CBD for daily treatment of depression, I generally recommend hemp-derived CBD because it is usually less expensive and you can obtain this without certification. However, because hemp-derived CBD is not regulated by the FDA, you must be very careful that you are getting a high-quality, full-spectrum, third-party-verified product. For the treatment of depression, I recommend 25 to 30 mg of CBD a day, which can be obtained by using CBD oil/tincture under the tongue, or CBD oil capsules. CBD, in general, does not immediately alleviate anxiety or depression, but rather taken daily for at least one to two weeks, it can start to affect some of the chemical signaling in the brain to help alleviate the anxiety component of depression, as well as the depression itself. Thus, don't expect to see improvement in symptoms right away.

Using Different Formulations for Depression

Almost as important as which strain of cannabis you use, or other factors such as the ratio of THC to CBD, is the formulation you use to treat depression. This is because different formulations have different onsets of actions and different durations. Unlike pain or headaches, which can come and go throughout the day, depression is usually there all the time. Thus, something that is going to last a long time is usually needed. However, some of the symptoms of depression, like acute anxiety or insomnia, may require medications that work quickly.

Pills or capsules (edibles) take longer to work (about an hour hour), but last longer in the body (up to eight hours) so some type of edible, either CBD-only or a cannabis edible, is usually needed for the treatment of depression. Depending on the state, some edibles may be available as an indica, sativa, or hybrid and may even be available in a specific strain.

Tinctures are liquids that come in droppers. You drop tincture under your tongue to allow for fast absorption rather than swallowing them directly. Tinctures take about thirty minutes to work, and last four to six hours. Tinctures are also slightly easier to titrate (adjust the dose) as they can be increased drop by drop. Finally, while this varies state by state, while most tinctures are extractions of primarily THC and CBD, some tinctures are available in sativa, indica, or hybrid strains, and some states sell extracts of the whole cannabis plant, so you can use a specific strain like the ones listed above. The role for tinctures in depression is more for some of the symptoms associated with depression, particularly insomnia and anxiety. Tinctures can be taken as needed for both of these conditions. As depression improves, these symptoms should hopefully abate.

Vape comes in the form of a concentrated liquid (called "**concentrate**") that is extracted from the marijuana plant, and usually heated so it can be inhaled. Vape also works very quickly (seconds to minutes), which is very beneficial for acute and severe symptoms, such as anxiety that is often associated with depression. However, it also doesn't last very long (an hour or so), meaning that any sedation or other effects will disappear quickly, so you can get back to your day. Almost all cannabis strains are available in vape or concentrate, so you don't have to smoke. You can choose one of those listed above (or similar) to start with. Since vape is most beneficial for anxiety or insomnia, starting with a hybrid or indica vape may be best.

General Recommendations for Depression

While depression is very common, everyone experiences depression quite differently. Similar to prescription medications, though without the side effects, using cannabinoids that are present in marijuana and hemp can help change the brain chemistry to treat depression as well as alleviate some of the associated symptoms. However, these changes don't usually occur immediately and can be substantially assisted with other forms of treatment such as counseling.

1. **Treat general depression by taking a high-dose CBD capsule pill or tincture every day.**
   Start with 25 to 30 mg of CBD a day in a pill/edible/capsule or tincture. This can either be a cannabis-derived CBD or pure-hemp-derived CBD. I generally recommend hemp-derived CBD as it is less expensive and easier to obtain, and because there is virtually no THC, it will not make you sleepy or high.

2. **Consider a sativa edible two to three times a day.**
   Because symptoms of depression are long lasting, edibles are best for daily depression, particularly those from a sativa strain. I recommend starting with an edible (mint, gummy, tablet, capsule)

derived from a sativa strain that has 5 mg of THC. Despite having THC, low doses of sativa edibles should not make you sleepy. Start with half a tablet two to three times a day, and increase by half a tablet each day or so to determine the amount of THC that helps with depression, but does not make you high.

3. **Address sleep issues by using nighttime cannabis with higher doses of THC, ideally with CBN.**
   Insomnia is a common symptom of depression, and the lack of a good night's sleep can contribute to further depression. Fortunately, cannabis is also very good at making people sleepy. In addition, to THC and CBD, there is also CBN, which stands for cannabinol. Like CBD, CBN is a nonpsychoactive cannabinoid, and CBN is particularly good for sleep. Five milligrams of CBN may be as effective as a 10-mg dose of diazepam (generic for Valium) for inducing sleep. There are several edibles and tinctures throughout the country that are available in a 1:1 ratio of CBN:THC. Some of these also contain terpenes and other natural components, such as organic chamomile or melatonin, that when combined with THC and CBN, can be quite effective to help induce sleep. Since tinctures only take about twenty to thirty minutes to work, and last about four to six hours, a 1:1 CBN:THC tincture is often a great place to start, as it can help you fall asleep and stay asleep. Check the milligrams per milliliter on the bottle to ensure you are getting the correct amount. For example, a 15 ml bottle with 50 mg of THC has over 3 mg THC per dropperful, so start with ½ dropperful 30 minutes before bedtime, and increase by a ¼ to ½ dropperful each evening until you are falling asleep easily and staying asleep.

   For patients who fall asleep just fine but get up early in the morning and can't fall back asleep ("terminal insomnia"), a pill or edible may be a better option. While pills or edibles take about an hour to start working, they last for six to eight hours. Start with an edible that contains 5 mg of THC, ideally from an indica strain. Some edibles will also contain components like melatonin to aid with sleep. Start with a half tablet for the first night or two. If that does not work, then increase the dose to a full tablet before bedtime. You can increase by half a tablet every two nights until you are staying asleep through the night.

For patients who have racing thoughts once they get in bed and turn off the lights, a vape or concentrate can also be used, since it works immediately. Indica strains, like GDP, usually work best. Start with one puff a few minutes before bedtime. You can increase by a puff every few minutes until you feel yourself getting sleepy. Patients who have problems both falling asleep and staying asleep (or terminal insomnia) can use both a vape right before bed to help them fall asleep, as well as an edible right before bedtime to keep them asleep. Finally, when using medical cannabis to help you sleep, do not forget about good sleeping habits (known as sleep hygiene): turn off the lights, do not watch TV in bed, and do not consume caffeine after 4:00 p.m.

4. **Use concentrate/vape for acute anxiety symptoms.**
Vape (also known as concentrate) is likely the best option for acute episodes of anxiety that are often associated with depression. A hybrid strain like Cannatonic that is low in THC may be particularly effective for daytime anxiety associated with depression. An indica strain like Granddaddy Purple has more THC and thus is stronger and more relaxing, but can also be sedating.

5. **Use nonmedicinal approaches in addition to cannabinoids.**
While beyond the scope of a book like this, it is worth mentioning that in addition to medicinal treatments for depression (including pharmaceuticals like Prozac, or natural products like medical cannabis), nonmedicinal treatments are also very effective. Meditation, yoga, and exercise are all examples of nonmedicinal treatments for depression. In addition, therapy with a trained professional (psychiatrist, psychologist, or counselor) is often very effective. Studies that have compared medicines to therapy usually

find them equally effective, and in fact, find the combination of both therapy and medication to be the most effective option.[5]

6. **Don't stop daily prescription medications right away.**
   Many patients I see with depression (as well as anxiety) are already taking prescription medications. While it might be wonderful if patients can treat their medical condition without prescriptions, I believe the goal should be to first improve symptoms. I recommend that patients generally stay on their medications until they are feeling better. While certain medicines that are supposed to be taken as needed, like benzodiazepines (Xanax/alprazolam, Valium/diazepam) and sedatives for sleep (Ambien/zolpidem), can be quickly replaced by cannabis, other medications meant to be taken daily, like SSRIs (Prozac/fluoxetine, Zoloft/sertraline, Lexapro/escitalopram) and bupropion (Wellbutrin) should not be stopped initially. Stopping these medicines immediately can make patients very sick. If you are using medical cannabis and CBD successfully, and are interested in trying to get off your daily prescription medication, please speak with your doctor first before doing so.

Chapter 15 Notes

1. Hasin, D. S., A. L. Sarvet, J. L. Meyers, et al. Epidemiology of Adult DSM-5 Major Depressive Disorder and Its Specifiers in the United States. *JAMA Psychiatry* 2018: 75(4), 336–346.

2. Ferguson, J. M. Depression: Diagnosis and Management for the Primary Care Physician. *Prim Care Companton J Clin Psychiatry* 2000 Oct: 2(5), 173–178.

3. Nutt, D., S. Wilson, and L. Paterson. Sleep disorders as core symptoms of depression. *Dialogues Clin Neurosci* 2008 Sep: 10(3), 329–336.

4. Demirkan, A., B. W. J. H. Penninx, K. Hek, et al. Genetic risk profiles for depression and anxiety in adult and elderly cohorts. *Mol Psychiatry* 2011 Jul: 16(7), 773–783.

5. Aherne, D., A. Fitzgerald, C. Aherne, et al. Evidence for the treatment of moderate depression: a systematic review. *Irish Journal of Psychological Medicine* 2017: 34(3), 197–204.

6. Regelson, W., J. R. Butler, J. Schulz, T. Kirk, L. Peek, M. L. Green, and M. O. Zalis. Delta 9-THC as an effective antidepressant and appetite-stimulating agent in advanced cancer patients. In M. C. Braude and S. Szara (Eds.), *The Pharmacology of Marihuana* (pp. 763–776). New York: Raven Press, 1976.

7. Turna, J., B. Patterson, and M. Van Ameringen. Is cannabis treatment for anxiety, mood, and related disorders ready for prime time? *Depression and Anxiety* 2017: 34(11), 1006–1017.

8. Hill, M. N., and B. B. Gorzalka. The endocannabinoid system and the treatment of mood and anxiety disorders. *CNS Neurol Disord Drug Targets* 2009 Dec: 8(6), 451–8.

9. de Mello Schier, A. R., N. P. de Oliveira Ribeiro, et al. Antidepressant-like and anxiolytic-like effects of cannabidiol: a chemical compound of Cannabis sativa. *CNS Neurol Disord Drug Targets* 2014: 13(6), 953–60.

10. Shannon, S., et al. Cannabidiol in Anxiety and Sleep: A Large Case Series. *Perm J* 2019: 23, 18–041.

Chapter 16:

How to Use Medical Cannabis and CBD for ADHD

What Is ADHD?

ADHD stands for attention deficit hyperactivity disorder, which is a disorder that commonly occurs in children in which they get symptoms including hyperactivity, impulsivity, and/or inattention. Not surprisingly, having these symptoms can affect a child's ability to function and develop properly in school or at home. More than 10% of school-age children can have ADHD, making it one of the more common disorders in childhood. For children, the diagnosis is made by having multiple symptoms of hyperactivity (difficulty sitting still or keeping quiet) or inattention (difficulty organizing tasks, staying focused) that occurs often and impairs the ability to function at school or home. Because ADHD is so common in children, it can also persist into adulthood. Adults can also be diagnosed with ADHD, and most (once diagnosed) report having had symptoms back in childhood. In addition to behavioral therapy, stimulant medications are usually used to treat children and adults. While this may seem counterintuitive, these medications appear to have the opposite affects in patients with ADHD.

Medical Marijuana for ADHD

The role for medical cannabis in ADHD is still evolving, but there is some evidence that it may be effective. THC is generally thought to be sedating, so one would think that cannabis might not be useful. However, a study analyzing postings on online discussion forums for ADHD patients found that 25% of patients indicated cannabis was helpful in treating their condition.[1] The mechanisms of stimulant prescription drugs in ADHD still remain unclear. One theory is that that ADHD may be due to a lack of dopamine, and THC in fact appears to increase levels of dopamine in the brain.[2] Another factor that may explain why the usually sedating THC may be helpful in treating ADHD is that different types of strains have different types of effects. While THC is generally sedating, sativa strains of cannabis, even with high amounts of THC, can be uplifting. In fact, the preferred strains for treating ADHD tend to be the sativa-leaning strains. Terpenes can also play a role in how cannabis affects the body, and thus how a particular strain of cannabis may be helpful in treating ADHD, despite some of the sedative effects usually associated with THC. Pinene is one of the more common terpenes found in cannabis and is particularly common in most sativa strains. Pinene is reported to increase alertness and elevate mood, which is not unlike prescription stimulants. While actual clinical studies are limited, there was one small trial (fifteen getting medication, fifteen getting placebo) of a prescription version of medical cannabis (Sativex, not available in the United States) in patients with ADHD.[3] The patients with ADHD taking medical cannabis had high scores on cognitive performance and activity levels, though because of the study's small size, the difference was not statistically significant. However, this study, along with some of the biologic effects of certain cannabis strains, does give a rationale for use of medical cannabis for treating patients with ADHD.

Further considerations in using medical cannabis to treat ADHD are the potentially synergistic effects of cannabis and stimulants when used simultaneously to treat ADHD. Both THC and stimulants such as methylphenidate can increase heart rate and blood pressure, and in fact when the two are taken together, they can have additive effects.[4] In fact, there is even a case report of a manic episode of a twenty-three-year-old male student using both methylphenidate and cannabis.[5] Thus, when using medical cannabis in combination with stimulant drugs, one should proceed with caution, starting with lower doses of THC.

Insomnia and Anxiety Are Both Common with ADHD

In addition to treating the specific symptoms of ADHD (hyperactivity, inattention), it is also important to treat some of the commonly associated symptoms of this disease. Fortunately, medical cannabis is particularly helpful in treating two of the most common symptoms associated with ADHD: insomnia and anxiety. Many children and adults with ADHD suffer from insomnia, including problems both falling asleep and staying asleep, which can have an impact performing at both work and school.[6] In addition, about half of patients with ADHD also have anxiety.[7] Even in patients without ADHD, anxiety and insomnia often occur together. However, the connection between these two conditions and ADHD is not entirely clear. One possible connection is related to changes in neurotransmitters, the chemical messengers in the brain that control thought and action, in which disturbances occur in all three conditions. Fortunately, both CBD and THC, like prescription medications used to treat anxiety and depression, can improve problems with neurotransmitters—though without the side effects that often occur with prescription drugs. Another possible connection between ADHD and both anxiety and insomnia is that the stimulant prescription medications used in ADHD can cause both anxiety and insomnia. Thus, another benefit of using medical cannabis in ADHD is that it can treat the symptoms of ADHD, while relieving (and not causing) anxiety and insomnia.

Strains for ADHD

Cannabis contains many different substances (called cannabinoids) that have medicinal properties. In addition to THC (the component that can make you "high") and CBD (which does not make you high), there are substances called terpenes that give marijuana its smell and flavor. The combination and proportion of cannabinoids and terpenes determine the effects of a particular cannabis strain on the body, with different strains of the cannabis plant having different proportions of these substances. The most common way of classifying different strains is dividing them into two categories: indica and sativa. Sativa strains are generally uplifting and energizing, while indica strains are generally more relaxing and sedating. As mentioned, pinene is a common terpene that is typically found in most sativa strains and (like prescription stimulants) has been reported to increase alertness and elevate mood. Thus, it is not surprising that sativa strains seem to be best for patients with ADHD. There are also hybrid strains, which can be balanced (half indica/half sativa) or more predominant in one or the other. Hybrid strains, even ones that are indica predominant, can be helpful in ADHD, especially when it comes to treating the anxiety or insomnia associated with ADHD. Anxiety and insomnia tend to respond better to indica strains. While the various strains and terpenes can be effective for ADHD and its associated symptoms, every patient is different, so it may take some trial and error to determine which strain is the right strain for you. A few strains that patients have successfully used for ADHD include the following:

Sour Diesel and **Green Crack.** Both of these strains are sativa strains that have a medium (15–20%) amount of THC, with very little (<1%) CBD and are preferred in patients that have ADHD. Both also contain the terpene caryophyllene, which is also useful in neve pain as well as depression.

Harle-Tsu is an indica-leaning hybrid. It has a very high CBD-to-THC ratio (up to 20:1), with less than 1% THC and about 10% CBD. Because of this, it is highly unlikely that Harle-Tsu will make you "high." It has myrcene, which can be relaxing, as well as terpinolene, which is a commonly used ingredient in soaps, perfumes, and lotions and can also be calming.

Gorilla Glue is an indica-predominant hybrid that is high in THC (24%) with low CBD. It contains multiple terpenes, including linalool, humulene, and caryophyllene. It can be most helpful when treating anxiety and insomnia.

CBD for ADHD

CBD is the nonpsychoactive cannabinoid in medical cannabis and is also found in hemp. It is known to be effective for anxiety, which as mentioned is commonly associated with ADHD. However, CBD's effects on ADHD alone are unclear. Unlike anxiety and epilepsy, where there is some research that supports the use of CBD in these conditions, research on cannabis for ADHD (above) is limited, and research on CBD alone is essentially nonexistent. Current reports of the benefit of using CBD alone in the treatment of ADHD is extremely limited and purely anecdotal. This doesn't mean that CBD is completely useless in the treatment of ADHD. There are two potential rationales for the use of CBD in ADHD. The first is the use of CBD to treat anxiety, which can be common in ADHD. The second is that CBD appears to counterbalance some of the unwanted effects (sedation, feeling "high") that is associated with THC. While cannabis strains contain both THC and CBD, many of the strains recommended for ADHD have low levels of CBD. Thus, the combination of both CBD- and THC-predominant strains may be effective.

While CBD-only products can be derived from either marijuana or hemp, I generally recommend hemp-derived CBD because it is usually less expensive, and you can obtain this without certification. However, because hemp-derived CBD is not regulated by the FDA, you must be very careful that you are getting a high-quality, full-spectrum, third-party-verified product. If you decide to try CBD for the treatment of ADHD, I recommend 25 to 30 mg of CBD a day, which can be obtained by using CBD oil/tincture under the tongue, or CBD oil capsules. CBD, in general, does not immediately alleviate anxiety, or symptoms of ADHD for that matter, but rather, taken daily for at least one to two weeks, it can start to affect some of the chemical signaling in the brain to help alleviate anxiety and possibly help with ADHD symptoms. Patients should not expect to see improvement in symptoms right away.

Using Different Formulations for ADHD

Almost as important as which strain of cannabis you use, or things like the ratio of THC to CBD, is the formulation you use to treat ADHD. This is because different formulations have different onsets of actions and different durations. Unlike pain or headaches, which can come and go throughout the day, ADHD is usually there all the time, and it usually affects people during the day when they are trying to work or pay attention in school. Thus, something that is going to last a long time, especially in the morning, is usually needed. However, while ADHD symptoms don't come on suddenly, faster-acting agents can be useful to start the day (since longer-lasting agents take longer to work), and faster-acting agents that can also be used to treat anxiety or insomnia may be needed as well.

Pills or capsules (edibles) take longer to work (about an hour), but last longer in the body (up to eight hours), so some type of edible is generally preferred for patients with ADHD, particularly in the morning. Depending on the state, some edibles may be available as an indica, sativa, or hybrid and may even be available in a specific strain.

Tinctures are liquids that come in droppers. You drop a tincture under your tongue to allow for fast absorption, rather than swallowing it directly. Tinctures take about thirty minutes to work and last four to six hours. Tinctures are also slightly easier to titrate (adjust the dose), as they can be increased drop by drop. Tinctures may also be easier for parents to give children who may not be able to swallow edibles and/or may not be appropriate for vaping. Finally, while this varies state by state, while most tinctures are extractions of primarily THC and CBD, some tinctures are available in sativa, indica, or hybrid strains, and some states sell extracts of the whole cannabis plant, so you can use a specific strain, like the ones listed above.

Vape commonly comes in the form of a concentrated liquid (called "**concentrate**") that is extracted from the marijuana plant, and usually heated so it can be inhaled. Vape also works very quickly (in seconds to minutes), which is very beneficial for acute and severe symptoms. However, it also doesn't last very long (an hour or so), meaning that vape alone is probably not practical for a condition that is always present, like ADHD. However, vape can be useful first thing in the morning, as well as for symptoms that require a faster onset of action, such as insomnia and anxiety. Almost all marijuana strains come in vape or concentrate, so you can choose one of those listed above (or similar) to start with. More than one vape may be needed, since sativa strains are best for ADHD symptoms, whereas hybrid strains would be more beneficial for anxiety or insomnia.

General Recommendations for ADHD

While ADHD is not uncommon, everyone experiences the effects of this condition differently. Similar to prescription medications (though without the side effects), using cannabinoids present in medical cannabis and hemp can help alter brain chemistry to help treat patients with ADHD, as well as some of the side effects associated with prescription medications used for this condition. Thus, it may take some adjustment to find the right strains, formulations, and doses that best treat your ADHD with or without prescription medications. The following are some general recommendations regarding how to get started:

1. **Use a sativa edible two to three times a day; tinctures may also work well.**

   Because ADHD is something that is constantly there, edibles can be taken a few times a day to control symptoms all day long. Because their effects may work similar to stimulants, sativa strains are best for ADHD patients. For example, several different companies in a variety of states make edibles (gummies, capsules, pills) that contain 5 mg of THC from a sativa strain. This can be helpful for ADHD, and despite having THC, should not make you sleepy. I recommend starting with half a tablet (2.5 mg) two to three times a day and increase by half a tablet each day/dose to determine the amount that helps with depression but does not make you high.

2. Use a sativa concentrate/vape to start the day.

Vape (also known as concentrate) works right away, so pairing it with the aforementioned recommended sativa edible, which can take up to an hour to work, is a great morning combination to start the day. Sour Diesel or Green Crack are sativa strains with a medium amount of THC. As with any vape, start with one puff to see how it affects your body. You should feel results within a few minutes. If you don't feel anything, you can try another puff. Eventually, you will figure out the number of puffs it takes to get you focused and allow you to concentrate, without feeling sleepy or high. For children, for whom vape may not be appropriate, or adults who prefer not to use vape, a sativa tincture can be a good alternative to a combination of vape and edible. Start with a small amount of a sativa tincture (2.5 mg) every four to six hours, and increase by a small amount each day until the desired effects are achieved, without feeling sedated or high.

3. Address sleep issues by using nighttime cannabis, such as indica-leaning hybrids with higher doses of THC.

As mentioned, insomnia is commonly associated with ADHD, and the lack of a good night's sleep can make ADHD symptoms worse. Fortunately, cannabis is also very good at making people sleepy. In addition to THC and CBD, there is also CBN, which stands for cannabinol. Like CBD, CBN is a nonpsychoactive cannabinoid, and CBN is particularly good for sleep. Five milligrams of CBN may be as effective as a 10-mg dose of diazepam (generic for Valium) for inducing sleep. There are several edibles and tinctures throughout the country that are available in a 1:1 ratio of CBN:THC. Some of these also contain terpenes and other natural components, such as organic chamomile or melatonin, that when combined with THC and CBN, can be quite effective to help induce sleep. Since tinctures only take about twenty to thirty minutes to work, and last about four to six hours, a 1:1 CBN:THC tincture is often a great place to start, as it can help you fall asleep and stay asleep. Check the milligrams per milliliter on the bottle to ensure you are getting the correct amount. For example, a 15-ml bottle with 50 mg of THC has over 3 mg of THC per dropperful, so start with ½ dropperful 30 minutes before bedtime, and increase by a ¼ to ½ dropperful each evening until you are falling asleep easily and staying asleep.

For patients who have more issues staying asleep than falling asleep, a pill or edible may be a better option. While pills or edibles take about an hour to start working, they last for six to eight hours. Start with an edible that contains 5 mg of THC, ideally from an indica strain. Some edibles will also contain components like melatonin to aid with sleep. Start with a half tablet for the first night or two. If that does not work, then increase the dose to a full tablet before bedtime. You can increase by half a tablet every two nights until you are staying asleep through the night.

For patients who have racing thoughts once they get in bed and turn off the lights, a vape or concentrate can also be used, since it works immediately. Indica strains or indica-leaning hybrids usually work best. Start with one puff a few minutes before bedtime. You can increase by a puff every few minutes until you feel yourself getting sleepy. Patients who have problems both falling asleep and staying asleep (or terminal insomnia) can use both a vape right before bed to help them fall asleep, as well as an edible right before bedtime, to keep them asleep. Finally, when using medical cannabis to help you sleep, do not forget about good sleeping habits (known as sleep hygiene): turn off the lights, do not watch TV in bed, and do not consume caffeine after 4:00 p.m.

4. **Use indica hybrids concentrate/vape for acute anxiety symptoms.** Vape (also known as concentrate) is also likely the best option for acute episodes of anxiety that are often associated with ADHD. An indica-leaning hybrid strain that is popular in patients with ADHD, such as Harle-Tsu, which is low in THC, may be particularly effective for daytime anxiety associated with ADHD. An indica strain like Gorilla Glue has more THC and thus is stronger and more relaxing but can also be sedating.

5. **Consider a trial of a high-dose CBD capsule pill or tincture every day.**

   Again, it is unclear whether or not CBD will help ADHD, but if symptoms aren't managed with cannabis and/or prescriptions, CBD might be an option. It can also alleviate unwanted effects of cannabis such as sedation and feeling "high." I recommend 25 to 30 mg of CBD a day in a pill/edible/capsule or tincture. This can either be a marijuana-derived CBD or pure-hemp-derived CBD, though I generally recommend hemp-derived CBD, as it is less expensive, easier to obtain, and because there is virtually no THC, it will not make you sleepy or high.

6. **Continue to use prescription medications, but use with caution.**

   Medical cannabis can be used as an alternative to prescription medications for ADHD or in addition to (adjunctive to) prescription medications, if they alone are not working. If you are taking ADHD medications but wish to switch to medical cannabis, I recommend doing this in consultation with the physician who prescribes these medications. I generally tell patients to continue their current medications and add low doses of cannabis first. Once some benefit can be appreciated by starting medical cannabis, prescriptions can by slowly decreased, while cannabis doses can be increased. As mentioned, since both THC and stimulants such as methylphenidate can increase heart rate and blood pressure, combing medical cannabis with prescription stimulants can have additive effects, so using both together should be done very cautiously. Starting with low doses of cannabis, closely monitoring symptoms as well as heart rate and blood pressure, and increasing cannabis doses slowly are advised.

7. **Don't forget about nonmedicinal approaches in addition to cannabinoids.**

   While beyond the scope of a book like this, it is worth mentioning that in addition to medicinal treatments for ADHD (including pharmaceuticals like Adderall, or natural products like cannabis), nonmedicinal treatments may also be effective. Nonpharmacologic therapies can either be behavioral, such as neurofeedback, cognitive training, cognitive behavioral therapy (CBT), or child or parent training, as well as dietary changes or use of supplements such as omega fatty acids.[8] Some patients may have the best benefit through a combination of prescriptions, cannabis and nonmedicinal approaches.

Chapter 16 Notes

1.   Mitchell, J. T., M. M. Sweitzer, et al. "I Use Weed for My ADHD": A Qualitative Analysis of Online Forum Discussions on Cannabis Use and ADHD. *PLoS One* 2016: 11(5), e0156614.

2.   Bloomfield, M. A. P., H. Ashok, N. D. Volkow, and O. D. Howes. The effects of Δ9-tetrahydrocannabinol on the dopamine system. *Nature* 2016 Nov 17: 539(7629), 369–377.

3.   Cooper, R. E., E. Williams, S. Seegobin, et al. Cannabinoids in attention-deficit/hyperactivity disorder: A randomised-controlled trial. *Eur Neuropsychopharmacol* 2017 Aug: 27(8), 795–808.

4.   Kollins, S. H., E. N. Schoenfelder, J. S. English, et al. An exploratory study of the combined effects of orally administered methylphenidate and delta-9-tetrahydrocannabinol (THC) on cardiovascular function, subjective effects, and performance in healthy adults. *J Subst Abuse Treat* 2015 Jan: 48(1), 96–103.

5.   Cinosi, E., M. Corbo, I. Matarazzo, et al. Cannabis and Methylphenidate-Induced Manic Symptoms. *J Clin Toxicol* 2015: 5, 3.

6.   Hvolby, A. Associations of sleep disturbance with ADHD: implications for treatment. *Atten Defic Hyperact Disord* 2015: 7(1), 1–18.

7.   Katzman, M. A., T. S. Bilkey, R. C. Pratap, et al. Adult ADHD and comorbid disorders: clinical implications of a dimensional approach. *BMC Psychiatry* 2017: 17, 302.

8.   Goode, A. P., R. R. Coeytaux, G. R. Maslow, et al. Nonpharmacologic Treatments for Attention-Deficit/Hyperactivity Disorder: A Systematic Review. *Pediatrics* 2018: 141(6), e2018.

Chapter 17:

How to Use Medical Cannabis and CBD for Chronic Pain

Different Types of Pain

Pain is complex. There are many types of pain that different people experience in a variety of ways. Patients who are having a heart attack often feel a "pressure," sometimes described as "an elephant sitting on my chest." Pain can be achy, stabbing, or burning. Different types of pain respond to different types of treatments. Fortunately, medical cannabis treats all types of pain.

There are generally two types of pain: acute and chronic. Acute pain is something that is severe and comes on suddenly. Pain after an injury or surgery is an acute pain. Chronic pain is unfortunately extremely common. It has been linked to a number of different physical and mental conditions, and also leads to increased health-care costs and lost productivity. In 2016, it was estimated that 20.4% of US adults suffered from chronic pain.[1] Chronic pain is often present all the time but usually waxes and wanes. Patients with chronic pain can get used to low levels of pain and are often able to function, but when pain is more severe, their activity can be severely limited, and quality of life severely impaired. There are many types of chronic pain, but for the purposes of using medical cannabis and CBD, we will describe two types: pain caused from inflammation and neuropathic pain, since their treatment is slightly different.

Inflammation is the body's natural healing process. When something gets injured or infected, the body starts a cascade of activity known as inflammation that fights infection, begins healing, and even wards off cancer. When you catch a cold and get a fever and runny nose, or when you sprain an ankle and get pain and swelling—that's inflammation. One of the consequences of inflammation is pain, which can actually be protective. Pain is telling your body to rest or not use your sprained ankle. However, chronically, inflammation can cause many problems, including pain. A common type of chronic pain is caused by inflammation is arthritis. Osteoarthritis (OA) is the wear and tear of bones that everyone gets over time as a result of aging. OA of the back, hips, and knees are most common, and patients often use anti-inflammatory medications, other pain medications, physical therapy, injections, and surgery. However, sometimes even these treatments do not help.

Neuropathic pain is pain caused by damaged nerves. The most common type of neuropathic pain is diabetic neuropathic pain, also called diabetic neuropathy. A combination of elevated blood sugar and impaired circulation causes damage to nerves, most commonly in the lower extremities. When nerves are damaged, they send incorrect signals, some of which are perceived as pain. Other types of nerve injury that can cause neuropathic pain include trauma, infection, or toxins. Neuropathy is not an uncommon side effect of chemotherapy used to treat cancer. Neuropathic pain is often described as burning or electric. It can also cause numbness and weakness.

Medical Cannabis for Pain

Fortunately, there is excellent evidence that medical cannabis is effective at treating pain. In 2017, the National Academies of Sciences reviewed all the available research regarding medical cannabis and its use in a variety of conditions. They found three areas in which they believed there was strong evidence to support the use of medical cannabis, one of which was chronic pain, particularly in those patients taking chronic opioid prescription medications.[2] The opioid epidemic is certainly a problem in our country, and cannabis may be one part of the solution. In fact, in one study that looked at prescription data for seniors taking pain medications, there was a reduction in the number of pain prescriptions in states where medical cannabis was legalized, with doctors writing 1,826 fewer pain prescriptions on average per year in states where medical cannabis was legal compared to doctors in nonlegal states.[3] Another study looking at deaths from opioid overdoses, from 1999 to 2010, showed that in states where medical cannabis was legal, there was a 24.8% lower rate of death from opiate overdoses than states where medical cannabis was not legalized.[4] In looking at actual clinical research, one analysis of multiple clinical trials[5] using medical cannabis for pain, patients experienced pain relief by 40% and a greater reduction in numerical pain scores. There were also several smaller trials that show that patients who take narcotics (opioids) for chronic pain can actually lower their opioid dose if they use medical cannabis.[6, 7] Medical cannabis has also been shown to be effective in at least one study in reducing pain after surgery.[8]

Strains for Pain

Cannabis contains many different substances (called cannabinoids) that have medicinal properties. In addition to THC (the component that can make you "high") and CBD (which does not make you high), there are substances called terpenes that give cannabis its smell and flavor. The combination and proportion of cannabinoids and terpenes will help determine which strains are best to treat your pain. While there are no randomized studies that have compared the various strains of cannabis plants and have determined which is the most effective for pain, patients who suffer from pain generally prefer indica-based strains, which also tend to be more relaxing and sedating. While indica-based strains have both THC and CBD, because THC is very important in treating pain, it is best to use a strain or product with at least some THC.

Two terpenes that can be beneficial for pain is beta-caryophyllene and myrcene. Beta-caryophyllene has a black pepper taste and smell and is helpful for both nerve pain and inflammation. Myrcene, which can also be found in hops, mango, and lemongrass, has muscle-relaxation properties in addition to helping with both pain and inflammation. While there are many strains that have been shown to be effective for pain, every patient is different, so it may take some trial and error to determine which strain is the right strain for you. A few strains that patients have successfully used for pain include the following:

Harlequin: A sativa-dominant hybrid with a higher CBD-to-THC ratio (5:2, with about 4–7% THC, 8–16% CBD), it is high in myrcene and can be effective for headaches without causing sedation and can actually be energizing. Thus, it is a popular daytime option for pain relief.

Jack Flash: Another sativa-dominant hybrid that is useful in managing pain during the day (despite being predominantly THC). It contains pinene, which is another terpene useful in pain. In addition to pain relief, Jack Flash is said to be neuroprotective and to have anti-inflammatory and antitumor effects as well.

White Widow: A hybrid strain which has about 20% THC and 1% CBD that works well for all types of pain and can improve mood and cause relaxation.

ACDC: Another balanced hybrid strain that is helpful for pain but known for its low levels of THC. It has the opposite ratio of White Widow, with a 20:1 CBD-to-THC ratio. Thus, this is one strain that will not make you high. Its predominant terpene is beta-myrcene, which can be helpful for pain.

CBD for Pain

While THC, the psychoactive component of medical cannabis, is extremely effective for pain, CBD can also be useful for pain, especially for pain caused by inflammation, such as OA. Research has shown CBD may have direct effects on inflammatory cells or may modulate the effects of certain pain receptors in the spinal cord.[9] While human studies are lacking, in an experimental model using rats, CBD has been shown to prevent pain caused by joint inflammation.[10]

CBD can be taken alone or combined with a low dose of THC and be quite effective for managing pain, especially during the day. Even though THC has some psychoactive properties, a low dose of THC will not make you "high" or sleepy. While having just a little THC appears to make CBD work better, pure CBD has anti-inflammatory and pain-relieving properties on its own. While you can use both marijuana-derived CBD, or hemp-derived CBD for pain and inflammation, I recommend hemp-derived CBD because it is generally less expensive, and you can obtain this without certification. However, because hemp-derived CBD is not regulated by the FDA, you must be careful that you are getting a high-quality, full-spectrum, third-party-verified product. For daily chronic pain, like OA, I recommend 25 to 30 mg of CBD a day, which can be obtained by using CBD oil/tincture under the tongue, or CBD oil capsules.

Using Different Formulations for Pain

Almost as important as which strain of cannabis you use, or the ratio of THC to CBD, is the formulation you use for pain control. This is because different formulations have different onsets of actions and different durations. Acute or severe pain requires a rapid onset of action (works in second or minutes), while chronic daily pain is best treated with something that lasts a long time.

Tinctures are liquids that come in droppers. You place drops of tincture under your tongue to allow for fast absorption, rather than swallowing them directly. Tinctures take about thirty minutes to work, and last four to six hours. Tinctures are also generally easier to titrate (slowly adjust) the dose, since doses can be increased drop by drop. Tinctures are often available in a variety of ratios of CBD to THC, which allow for further customization of balancing pain relief and sedation, or getting "high." In addition, while this varies state by state, though most tinctures are extractions of primarily THC and CBD, some tinctures are available in sativa, indica, or hybrid strains, and some states sell extracts of the whole cannabis plant, so you can use a specific strain like the ones listed above.

Pills or capsules (edibles) take a bit longer to work (one to two hours) but last longer in the body (up to eight hours), so they can be an excellent choice for constant pain, especially for patients trying to get off long-acting narcotics, like OxyContin. Depending on the state, some edibles may be available as an indica, sativa, or hybrid and may even be available in a specific strain.

Vape comes in the form of a concentrated liquid (called "**concentrate**") that is extracted from the marijuana plant, and usually heated so it can be inhaled. Vape also works very quickly (seconds to minutes), which is very beneficial for acute and severe pain. However, it also doesn't last very long (an hour or so), meaning that any sedation or other effects will disappear quickly, so you can get back to your day. Almost all cannabis strains come in vape or concentrate, so you can choose one of those listed above (or similar) to start with.

Topical formulations of medical cannabis come in salves and balms and can be very effective for local pain. Despite having a high amount of THC, because they are applied to the skin, very little is absorbed in the bloodstream, and thus topical formulations have no psychoactive properties. Balms or creams only last a few hours and thus should be applied regularly. They are particularly good for pain when it occurs on a specific area of the body, such as low-back pain. One downside of topical formulations is that they tend to be much more expensive than other formulations. Spreading a topical over your entire body can be quite expensive, so I generally recommend topicals only for localized pain.

General Recommendations for Acute and Chronic Pain

It is difficult to recommend a specific pain regimen in a handout or book because every patient's pain is so different, and every patient will react somewhat differently to different strains, formulations, and amounts of THC. However, to provide you some guidance, below are some general recommendations for treating pain. Please remember that since the general recommendation for using medical cannabis it to "start low, go slow," you will likely need some patience when using medical cannabis to treat pain, especially chronic pain.

1. **Take a daily, high-dose CBD capsule pills or tincture daily.**
CBD has anti-inflammatory properties, which can in turn reduce
pain. Thus, any patient with chronic pain should take CBD
daily, not only to treat pain but to treat the cause of the pain in a
preventative manner. This is especially true for chronic pain from
inflammation, such as OA. CBD can also improve range of motion
and decrease scar tissue. Start with 25 to 30 mg of CBD daily in
either a pill/capsule or tincture. This can either be a cannabis-
derived CBD or a full-spectrum hemp-derived CBD. I generally
recommend hemp-derived CBD, as it is less expensive, easier to
obtain, and because there is virtually no THC, it will not make
you sleepy or high.

2. **For chronic pain, use edibles or tincture several times a day
with a 2:1 or 1:1 ratio of CBD to THC for daily pain, either
regularly or as needed.**
Patients with chronic pain, usually have some pain all the time
and take daily pain medications. Thus, regular use of pills/edible
or tinctures should help keep this pain at bay. This will usually be
about two to four times a day, depending which ones you use and
how severe your pain is.

   While edibles and tinctures come in a variety of ratios of CBD
to THC (14:1, 4:1, 1:1, 1:4, et cetera), since I recommend that
patients take higher doses of daily CBD, I have found it much easier
(and less expensive) for patients to stick with 2:1 or 1:1 products.
Since pills and tinctures are often reconstituted with terpenes added
back, choose products specifically designed for pain, which have
terpenes such as beta-caryophyllene and myrcene. While each state
is different, some companies make edibles and tinctures that are
either sativa, indica, or hybrid, and some companies even make
strain-specific products, so you can use one of the strains listed above.
Start with approximately 0.5 to 1 mg of THC for the first dose. You
can figure out how much THC is in one pill or one dropperful of
tincture by looking at the package. For example, in a 2:1 tincture

that comes in a 15-ml bottle with 300 mg cannabinoids, half a dropperful (0.5 ml or 10 drops) contains 10 mg of cannabinoids. So 3 drops will be about 2 mg of CBD and 1 mg THC. You can start with about 5 drops (1–2mg of THC) each day, or even with each dose, and then slowly increase the amount of THC drop by drop until you get the desired amount of pain relief without side effects. Edibles are easier to dose because the milligrams are stated on the package, and you can usually easily cut an edible in one-half or one-quarter to achieve your desired dose. Most patients achieve good results at 2 to 15 mg of THC per dose.

3. **Use vape for severe, acute pain.**

Most patients with chronic pain have breakthrough pain that can be acute. Thus, something that works quickly like vape is needed. Whereas CBD is taken every day, and pills and tincture mixes of THC and CBD are taken regularly, vape can be used for when pain flares up or is severe. Be sure to use a vape that is a concentrate from a cannabis strain that is particularly good for pain. White Widow, Harlequin, Jack Flash, and ACDC are just a few strains found to be helpful for pain. Start with one puff at the onset of pain, and wait a few minutes to determine its effect on your pain. Slowly increase your dose by one puff at a time. Eventually, you will determine the number of puffs it takes to relieve acute pain without getting sleepy or high.

4. **Use topical preparations for localized pain, or in the area of worst pain when multiple areas exist.**

Topical balms and ointments can be very effective for patients with localized pain (i.e., pain in once specific area). It can either be used in addition to the regimen above or used exclusively for localized pain. For example, in a patient who only has shoulder pain, especially after activity, a cannabis cream prior to activity may be all that is needed. In contrast, in a patient with severe osteoarthritis in their back, shoulders, hands, but that is particularly worse in their knees, can use daily CBD, tinctures, or edibles throughout the day for chronic pain, vape for breakthrough pain (as described above), as well as topical cream on their knees two to three times a day, since this is where pain is the worst.

5. **Address sleep issues related to pain.**
   Many patients with pain also have sleep issues. Having chronic pain can make it difficult to sleep. Fortunately, cannabis is also particularly good at making people sleepy. In addition to THC and CBD, there is also CBN, which stands for cannabinol. Like CBD, CBN is a nonpsychoactive cannabinoid, and CBN is particularly good for sleep. Five milligrams of CBN may be as effective as a 10-mg dose of diazepam (generic for Valium) for inducing sleep. There are both tinctures and edibles that come in 1:1 CBN:THC ratios. Some also contain natural ingredients such as chamomile and melatonin that can be quite effective to help induce sleep. In addition, some tinctures and edibles contain THC from indica strains, and in some states, you can get tinctures as a whole-plant extract of a particular strain. Since tinctures only take about twenty to thirty minutes to work and last about four to six hours, an indica-based tincture, especially one containing CBN, is often a great place to start as it can help patients both fall asleep and stay asleep. Start with a ½ dropperful thirty minutes before bedtime, and increase by a ¼ to ½ dropperful each evening until you are falling asleep easily and staying asleep. For patients who have more issues staying asleep than falling asleep, a pill or edible may be a better option. While pills or edibles take about an hour to start working, they last six to eight hours. A 5-mg THC edible, particularly if it is an indica strain and/or contains CBN, would be another good option. Start with a half tablet for the first night or two. If that doesn't work, then go up to the one full tablet. You can increase by half a tablet every two nights until you are staying asleep.

6. **For those on daily opioids, continue them, at least initially.**
   Many patients with chronic pain use narcotics or opioids to control their pain and are seeking medical cannabis as an alternative. The

opioid crisis in the United States is serious. Opioids can be dangerous, as hundreds of patients die each day from overdoses. Opioids also have many side effects, including severe constipation and nausea. Fortunately, cannabinoids are synergistic with opioids, and research has proven that patients at a minimum can lower their opioid dose when using medical marijuana. However, the goal of medical cannabis should be pain control first, followed by lowering opioid doses. In addition, opioids are highly addictive, and stopping opioids too quickly can lead to withdrawal symptoms. Many patients on opioids take both long-acting pain meds (Oxycontin, fentanyl patch) and short-acting pain medications (Percocet). In addition, I have found that most patients on regular narcotics are still in pain despite taking these medications regularly. Thus, my recommendation for patients who are already using opioids is to start with the general recommendations described above for acute and chronic pain, while continuing to take their current dose of narcotic medications. If patients find their pain is well controlled on the combination of cannabis and opioids, they can try a lower dose of their short-acting narcotics (i.e., one Percocet instead of two) when using their daily or breakthrough cannabis pain medication. The lowering of opioid medications should be done very slowly. In addition, as opioid doses are lowered, patients may find they need to increase their cannabis dosages. Once patients are on a daily cannabis regimen that controls their pain and have lowered their total opioid dose, especially if they remain on any long-acting narcotic medications, they can then slowly taper off their opioid medicines to avoid withdrawal symptoms. Since this can be quite complex and lead to severe symptoms, I highly recommend doing this in consultation with the physician prescribing the narcotics, even if they are not the provider who certified the patient for medical cannabis.

7. **High doses and faster onset may be needed for nonresponders.** Most patients achieve good pain control between 2 to 15 mg of THC per dose. For a 2:1 tincture, that could be between one-quarter

to two full dropperfuls. However, for a small percentage of patients, low-to-moderate-dose cannabis (≤60mg of THC daily) is not sufficient. If patients get no response in a few weeks, they can switch to higher-dose products that contain more THC. One example of a concentrated product is Rick Simpson's Oil, or RSO. Often a drop as small as a grain of rice has more THC than several droppers of tincture. This should be used carefully because of the high potency and the fact that the small size of the dose can lead to significant dose variability. In addition, patients who may be reluctant to use vape should strongly consider vape if their initial response to edibles and tinctures is not sufficient.

1

Chapter 17 Notes

1. Dahlhamer, J., J. Lucas, C. Zelaya, et al. Prevalence of Chronic Pain and High-Impact Chronic Pain Among Adults—United States, 2016. *MMWR Morb Mortal Wkly Rep* 2018: 67, 1001–1006.

2. National Academies of Sciences, Engineering, and Medicine. The Health Effects of Cannabis and Cannabinoids: The Current State of Evidence and Recommendations for Research. Washington, DC: The National Academies Press, 2017.

3. Bradford, A. C., and W. D. Bradford. Medical marijuana laws reduce prescription medication use in Medicare part D. *Health Affairs* 2016: 35(7), 1230–1236.

4. Bachhuber, M. A., B. Saloner, C. O. Cunningham, et al. Medical Cannabis Laws and Opioid Analgesic Overdose Mortality in the United States, 1999-2010. *JAMA Intern Med* 2014: 174(10), 1668–1673.

5. Whiting, P. F., R. F. Wolff, S. Deshpande, et al. Cannabinoids for Medical Use: A Systematic Review and Meta-analysis. *JAMA* 2015 Jun 23–30: 313(24), 2456–73.

6. Boehnke, K. F., E. Litinas, and D. J. Clauw. Medical Cannabis Use Is Associated With Decreased Opiate Medication Use in a Retrospective Cross-Sectional Survey of Patients With Chronic Pain. *J Pain* 2016 Jun: 17(6), 739–44.

7. Abrams, D. I., P. Couey, S. B. Shade, et al. Cannabinoid-opioid interaction in chronic pain. *Clin Pharmacol Ther* 2011 Dec: 90(6), 844–51.

8. Holdcroft, A., M. Maze, C. Doré, S. Tebbs, and S. Thompson. A multicenter dose-escalation study of the analgesic and adverse effects of an oral cannabis extract (Cannador) for postoperative pain management. *Anesthesiology* 01 May 2006: 104(5), 1040–1046.

9. Xiong, W., C. Tanxing, et al. Cannabinoids suppress inflammatory and neuropathic pain by targeting α3 glycine receptors. *J Exp Med* 2012 Jun 4: 209(6), 1121–1134.

10. Philpott, H. T., M. O'Brien, and J. J. McDougall. Attenuation of early phase inflammation by cannabidiol prevents pain and nerve damage in rat osteoarthritis. *Pain* 2017: 158(12), 2442–2451.

Chapter 18:

How to Use Medical Cannabis and CBD for Headaches and Migraines

Different Types of Pain, Different Types of Headaches

Pain is complex. Pain can be achy, stabbing, or burning. Different types of pain respond to different types of treatments. Fortunately, medical cannabis treats many types of pain, and using medical cannabis for headache pain is actually not too complex. There are generally two types of pain: acute and chronic. Acute pain is something that is severe and comes on suddenly. Pain after an injury or surgery is an acute pain. Chronic pain is often there all the time but usually waxes and wanes. Headaches are tricky, because when they come on, they can be very acute. However, some people have headaches almost all the time (often referred to as chronic daily headaches), so there is a chronic pain element of their headaches.

To add to the confusion, while headaches cause pain, there are different types of headaches with different types of causes. In addition, the causes of most kinds of headaches are not clearly understood. While there are many types of headaches, which sometimes overlap, to keep things simple for treatment purposes, I will divide headaches into to two categories: migraine and typical headache.

The mechanisms that cause migraine headaches are not entirely clear. Theories include a mix of vascular, muscle, and nervous system components. Inflammation may also play a role. The good news is that cannabis has been shown to help with migraine headaches. While all migraine headaches do not present like a typical migraine, a typical migraine is described as coming on suddenly and severely, usually on one side of the head, where the patient is bothered by light and sound. Migraines are often accompanied by nausea. By contrast, a more typical headache (sometimes called tension headache), usually occurs on both sides of the head (usually in the front) and is often provoked by stress. While typical headaches are not usually as severe as migraines, they can still be very painful and debilitating. In addition, migraines tend to last hours to days, where typical headaches can occur on a daily basis, becoming more chronic, and are often referred to as chronic daily headaches.

The most common treatments for both types of headaches include over-the-counter-pain medicines such as nonsteroidal anti-inflammatory medications (NSAID's) like ibuprofen and naproxen, as well as acetaminophen (Tylenol), sometimes with caffeine (Excedrin). While these medications can be effective, long-term use can be problematic. NSAIDs can cause stomach bleeding and kidney issues. Acetaminophen used in high doses can cause liver problems. A migraine-specific class of prescription medications called the "triptans," is very effective for some patients if taken right at the onset of a migraine. Unfortunately, they do not work for all patients.

Medical Cannabis for Headaches and Migraines

Ultimately, the main symptom for both headaches and migraines is pain. There is robust evidence that medical cannabis is effective at treating pain. In 2017, the National Academies of Sciences report that reviewed all the available research regarding medical cannabis found that one of the three areas in which there was strong evidence to support the use of medical cannabis was chronic pain.[1] One analysis of multiple clinical trials[2] using medical cannabis for pain, showed that patients experienced pain relief by 40% and a greater reduction in numerical pain scores. Several smaller trials showed that patients who take narcotics (opioids) for chronic pain can actually lower their opioid dose if they use medical cannabis.[3, 4] In addition, medical cannabis has also been shown to be effective in at least one study in reducing pain after surgery.[5]

In regard to headache use specifically, the research is less substantial but certainly exists. In a large survey of medical cannabis users, about a quarter of the patients were using medical cannabis to treat headache.[6] A review of the literature from 2018 found several studies indicating that medical cannabis could be effective for headache and migraine.[7] In addition to its general pain-relieving ability, and limited research supporting its use for all types of headaches, medical cannabis may be particularly useful for migraine headaches. Studies suggest that patients with migraines may suffer from low levels or a deficiency of our own natural cannabinoids (endocannabinoids).[8] Thus, supplementation of low levels of endocannabinoids by plant-based cannabinoids (phyto-cannabinoids) makes logical sense and is essentially treating the disease and not just the symptoms.

Strains for Headaches and Migraines

The cannabis plant contains many different substances (called cannabinoids) that have medicinal properties. In addition to THC (the component that can make you "high") and CBD (which does not make you high), there are substances called terpenes that give cannabis its smell and flavor. The combination and proportion of cannabinoids and terpenes will help determine which strains are best to treat your headache. Beta-caryophyllene is a terpene that has a black pepper taste and smell and is helpful for neurologic pain, as well as inflammation. Myrcene is another terpene that can also be found in hops, mango, and lemongrass, and it has muscle-relaxation properties in addition to helping with pain. Limonene is also found in citrus fruits and may be beneficial for anxiety, pain, and inflammation. While strains with these terpenes can be effective for headaches, every patient is different, so it may take some trial and error to determine which strain is the right strain for you. A few strains that patients have successfully used for headache include the following:

Harlequin: A sativa-dominant hybrid with a higher CBD-to-THC ratio (5:2, with about 4–7% THC, 8–16% CBD), it is high in myrcene and can be effective for headaches without causing sedation and can actually be energizing. Thus, it is a popular daytime option.

White Widow: A balanced hybrid strain that has about 20% THC and 1% CBD. It works well for all types of pain and can improve mood and cause relaxation.

ACDC: Another balanced hybrid strain that is helpful for pain but known for its low levels of THC. It has the opposite ratio of White Widow, with 20:1 CBD-to-THC ratio. Thus, this is one strain that will not make you high. Its predominant terpene is beta-myrcene, which can be helpful for pain. It is also helpful for anxiety and depression, which may be triggers for headaches.

Northern Lights: A myrcene-heavy indica strain that is particularly good for acute pain. It has a medium amount (14–19%) of THC, and very little (l<1%) CBD.

Bubba Kush: Another indica strain high in caryophyllene, myrcene. It also has some limonene. It can be very sedating and tranquilizing. It also has a medium amount (14–19%) of THC, and very little (l<1%) CBD.

CBD for Headaches and Migraines

While THC, the psychoactive component of medical cannabis, can be effective for headaches, CBD may also be useful in headaches and migraines. While the cause for both typical headaches and migraine headaches are unknown, stress and inflammation both may play roles, and CBD is particularly good for reducing stress and can act as an anti-inflammatory.[9] In addition, CBD has been found in mostly non-human studies to be neuroprotective, which means that it has been shown to help lessen the effects of damaged brain cells in conditions such as stroke, including the possibility of helping the growth of new brain cells.[10] Whether or not neuroprotection is important for headaches and migraines is unclear. Finally, brain activity may be an important factor in headaches and migraines. While there is limited research on CBD alone on headaches and migraines, there is a substantial amount of research on high-dose CBD in the treatment of seizures. In fact, Epidiolex is a cannabis-based, CBD-only product that is FDA approved for the treatment of seizures.[11] There is some thought that the causes of migraines and seizures are similar, and some prescription seizure medications have been used with success in treating migraines. Whether this translates to using either prescription Epidiolex or hemp-derived CBD is unclear. However, this further strengthens the rationale for trying CBD in the treatment of both migraine and tension headaches.

CBD can be taken alone or combined with a very low dose of THC and be quite effective for managing headaches, especially during the day. Even though THC has some psychoactive properties, a very low dose of THC should not make you "high" or sleepy. While you can use both cannabis-derived CBD or hemp-derived CBD for daily use for the prevention of headaches and migraines, I recommend hemp-derived CBD because it is generally less expensive and you can obtain this without certification. However, because hemp-derived CBD is not regulated by the FDA, you must be very careful that you are getting a high-quality, full-spectrum, third-party-verified product. For chronic daily headaches, or for the prevention of migraines, I recommend 25 to 30 mg of CBD a day, which can be taken by using CBD oil/tincture under the tongue, or CBD oil capsules.

Using Different Formulations for Headaches and Migraine

Almost as important as which strain of cannabis you use, or the ratio of THC to CBD, is the formulation you use to treat headaches and migraines. This is because different formulations have different onsets of actions and different durations. Acute or severe pain, especially at first onset of a migraine, requires a rapid onset of action (working in seconds or minutes), while chronic headache is best treated with something that lasts a long time.

Tinctures are liquids that come in droppers. You drop a tincture under your tongue to allow for fast absorption rather than swallowing it directly. Tinctures take about thirty minutes to work, and last four to six hours, so they can be excellent for regular chronic headaches.

Tinctures are also slightly easier to titrate (adjust the dose), as they can be increased drop by drop. Finally, while this varies state by state, while most tinctures are extractions of primarily THC and CBD, some tinctures are available in sativa, indica, or hybrid strains, and some states sell extracts of the whole cannabis plant, so you can use a specific strain like the ones listed above.

Pills or capsules (edibles) take a bit longer to work (one to two hours), but last longer in the body (up to eight hours), so they can be an excellent choice for constant pain. Depending on the state, some edibles may be available as an indica, sativa, or hybrid and may even be available in a specific strain.

Vape comes in the form of a concentrated liquid (called "**concentrate**") that is extracted from the cannabis plant, and usually heated so it can be inhaled. Vape also works very quickly (seconds to minutes), which is very beneficial for acute and severe pain, including at the onset of a migraine. However, it also doesn't last very long (an hour or so), meaning that any sedation or other effects will disappear quickly, so you can get back to your day. Almost all cannabis strains come in vape or concentrate, so you can choose one of those listed above (or similar) to start with.

General Recommendations for Migraine and Headaches

While migraine headaches and typical headaches/chronic daily headaches are different in both their cause and how patients are affected, the approach to using medical cannabis and CBD is not all that different, though the relative importance of the different components of the following regimen may vary, depending on how a patient individually experiences headache. For example, nausea is more frequently associated with migraine headaches, so patients who don't have nausea can skip that recommendation, regardless of the type of headache they get.

1. **Prevent migraine or chronic daily headaches by taking a high-dose CBD capsule pill or tincture (with or without a small dose of THC) every day.**

   Given their role in seizures and anxiety, as well as having some anti-inflammatory properties which may be relevant in headaches, I recommend that any patient with migraines or chronic daily headaches take CBD daily, not so much to treat the headaches (though there will likely be some benefit), but rather to be used in more of a preventative manner. Start with 25 to 30 mg of CBD a day in a pill/edible/capsule or tincture. This can either be a cannabis-derived CBD or pure-hemp-derived CBD. I generally recommend hemp-derived CBD, as it is less expensive and easier to obtain, and because there is virtually no THC, it will not make you sleepy or high.

2. **Address sleep issues by using nighttime cannabis with higher doses of THC.**

   Many patients with headaches also have sleep issues, and the lack of a good night's sleep can contribute to headaches. Fortunately, cannabis is also very good at making people sleepy. Patients who also have sleeping issues should take a product in the evening that is particularly effective for sleep. In addition to THC and CBD, there is also CBN, which stands for cannabinol. Like CBD, CBN is a nonpsychoactive cannabinoid, and CBN is particularly good for sleep. Five milligrams of CBN may be as effective as a 10-mg dose of diazepam (generic for Valium) for inducing sleep. There are both tinctures and edibles that come in 1:1 CBN:THC ratios. Some also contain natural ingredients, such as chamomile and melatonin, that can be quite effective to help induce sleep. In addition, some tinctures and edibles contain THC from indica strains, and in some states, you can get tinctures as a whole-plant extract of a particular strain.

3. **Use concentrate/vape at the onset of a migraine or severe headache.**

   Patients with migraines often have what known as an "aura," when they can tell a migraine is coming. Patients with typical headaches may also have severe headaches that come on strong, seemingly out of nowhere. In both instances, something that works quickly like vape is needed. Whereas CBD is taken every day, and pills or tinctures that combine THC and CBD can be regularly for symptoms, vape should be used at the onset of a migraine and/ or when headache pain is severe. Use a vape that is a concentrate from a cannabis strain that is particularly good for headaches (described above), which include White Widow, Harlequin, ACDC, and Northern Lights. When dosing a vape, start with one puff. Wait a few minutes until you feel an effect. You can increase the dose slowly, one puff at a time, until you feel relief from your headache, without feeling sleepy or high.

4. **Take pills/edibles or tincture several times a day with a 2:1 or 1:1 ratio of CBD to THC for constant headache pain, either regularly or as needed.**

   Some patients, both with migraines and typical headaches, have headaches that last all day. Those with chronic daily headaches can have headaches most or every day. Thus, regular use of pills/ edible or tinctures can help keep these types of headaches under control. Edibles last six to eight hours, and tinctures last four to six hours, so patients may need to take these remedies a few times a day. While edibles and tinctures come in a variety of ratios of CBD to THC (14:1, 4:1, 1:1, 1:4, et cetera), since I recommend that patients take higher doses of daily CBD, I have found it much easier (and less expensive) for patients to stick with 2:1 or 1:1 products. Since pills and tinctures are often reconstituted with terpenes added back, chose products specifically designed for pain, which have terpenes such as beta-caryophyllene and myrcene. While each state is different, some companies make edibles and tinctures that are either sativa, indica, or hybrid, and some companies even make strain-specific products, so you can use one of the strains listed above. Start with approximately 0.5 to 1 mg of THC for the first dose. You can figure out how much THC is in one pill or one dropperful of tincture by looking at the package. For example, a 2:1 tincture that comes in a 15-ml bottle with 300 mg cannabinoids, half a dropperful (0.5 ml or 10 drops) contains 10 mg of cannabinoids. So three drops will be about 2 mg of CBD and 1 mg THC. You can start with about 5 drops (1–2 mg of THC) each day, or even with each dose, and then slowly increase the amount of THC drop by drop until you get the desired amount of pain relief without side effects. Edibles are easier to dose because the milligrams are stated on the package, and you can usually easily cut an edible in half or in a quarter to achieve your desired dose. Most patients achieve good results at 2 to 15 mg of THC per dose.

Chapter 18 Notes

1. National Academies of Sciences, Engineering, and Medicine. The Health Effects of Cannabis and Cannabinoids: The Current State of Evidence and Recommendations for Research. Washington, DC: The National Academies Press, 2017.

2. Whiting, P. F., R. F. Wolff, S. Deshpande, et al. Cannabinoids for Medical Use: A Systematic Review and Meta-analysis. *JAMA* 2015 Jun 23–30: 313(24), 2456–73.

3. Boehnke, K. F., E. Litinas, and D. J. Clauw. Medical Cannabis Use Is Associated With Decreased Opiate Medication Use in a Retrospective Cross-Sectional Survey of Patients With Chronic Pain. *J Pain* 2016 Jun: 17(6), 739–44.

4. Abrams, D. I., P. Couey, S. B. Shade, et al. Cannabinoid-opioid interaction in chronic pain. *Clin Pharmacol Ther* 2011 Dec: 90(6), 844–51.

5. Holdcroft, A., M. Maze, C. Doré, S. Tebbs, and S. Thompson. A multicenter dose-escalation study of the analgesic and adverse effects of an oral cannabis extract (Cannador) for postoperative pain management. *Anesthesiology* 01 May 2006: 104(5), 1040–1046.

6. Baron, E. P., P. Lucas, J. Eades, and O. Hogue. Patterns of medicinal cannabis use, strain analysis, and substitution effect among patients with migraine, headache, arthritis, and chronic pain in a medicinal cannabis cohort. *J HEADACHE PAIN* 2018: 19(1), 37.

7. Baron, E. P. Medicinal Properties of Cannabinoids, Terpenes, and Flavonoids in Cannabis, and Benefits in Migraine, Headache, and Pain: An Update on Current Evidence and Cannabis Science. *Headache* 2018: 58(7), 1139–1186.

8. Russo, E. B. Clinical endocannabinoid deficiency reconsidered: current research supports the theory in migraine, fibromyalgia, irritable bowel, and other treatment-resistant syndromes. *Cannabis and cannabinoid research* 2016: 1(1), 154–165.

9. Xiong, W., C. Tanxing, et al. Cannabinoids suppress inflammatory and neuropathic pain by targeting α3 glycine receptors. *J Exp Med* 2012 Jun 4; 209(6), 1121–1134.

10. Campos, A. C., M. V. Fogaça, A. B. Sonego, and F. S. Guimarães. Cannabidiol, neuroprotection and neuropsychiatric disorders. *Pharmacol Res* 2016 Oct: 112, 119–127.

11. Epidiolex package insert. https://www.accessdata.fda.gov/drugsatfda_docs/label/2018/210365lbl.pdf. Accessed 12/14/2019.

Chapter 19:

How to Use Medical Cannabis and CBD for Dementia and Alzheimer's Disease

What Are Dementia and Alzheimer's Disease?

As we get older, there are naturally occurring changes in the brain. We start to lose memory, especially short-term memory. Age-associated changes in the brain are not always bad. In fact, as the brain ages, creativity can actually increase. However, when one's memory and mental ability decline significantly enough to interfere with daily life, this is called dementia. Dementia is not a normal part of aging, and there are many causes of dementia. Alzheimer's disease or Alzheimer's dementia is the most common cause of dementia. In 2011, there were 4.5 million seniors over the age of sixty-five living with Alzheimer's dementia.[1]

In Alzheimer's disease the brain is damaged when certain proteins lead to inflammation and deposits in the brain that in turn lead to plaques and webs of tissue called neurofibrillary tangles.[2] These tangles cause the clinical features in Alzheimer's dementia, which initially includes short-term memory loss but eventually leads to behavioral changes. Even in early Alzheimer's, executive function and judgment can be impaired, but later in the disease, there are disturbances in behavior, which can include agitation, aggression, wandering, and even psychosis. Other types of dementia exist but are caused by something other than neurofibrillary tangles. For example, vascular dementia is caused by decreased blood flow to the brain and is the second most common type of dementia.[3] While there are certainly differences between Alzheimer's disease and other forms of dementia, all can be characterized by memory loss and behavior changes, which medical cannabis can help with. Thus, for the purposes of this chapter, we will discuss medical cannabis and CBD treatment of Alzheimer's disease and other dementias collectively.

Medical Cannabis for Dementia and Alzheimer's Disease

Medical cannabis for the treatment of Alzheimer's disease and other forms of dementia continue to evolve as we begin to have better understanding of both the disease process itself, as well as how cannabis might be able to help. Use of medical cannabis to treat these conditions is not uncommon, and Alzheimer's disease is a qualifying condition for use of medical marijuana in thirteen states. There are essentially two ways to think about medical cannabis and its use in Alzheimer's disease and dementia: treating the underlying condition and treating the symptoms.

In terms of treating the underlying condition, there is very limited evidence that cannabis can treat the underlying disease, or the primary memory deficit seen in all forms of dementia. There is one study, using cells in a test tube, that demonstrated that small amounts of THC might inhibit production of beta amyloid, which is the key component of the neurofibrillary tangles seen in Alzheimer's disease.[4] However, this is far from clear evidence that cannabis can help the underlying process, either in prevention or treatment, of Alzheimer's disease or other forms of dementia.

The case for treating the symptoms of Alzheimer's disease and dementia is far more compelling. Symptoms other than memory and cognition that are associated with brain disorders are called neuropsychiatric symptoms. These neuropsychiatric symptoms commonly occur with all types of dementia and include agitation, aggression, wandering, apathy, sleep disorders, depression, anxiety, psychosis, and eating disorders.[5] One recent study from Canada that reviewed all of the available research looking into the benefit of medical cannabis for dementia concluded that medical cannabis may be effective for treating the following symptoms: agitation, disinhibition, irritability, aberrant motor behavior, and nocturnal behavior disorders, as well as aberrant vocalization and resting care.[6] The study noted that most of the studies were small and limited in their scope and design, but did provide supportive evidence for the use of medical cannabis for the treatment of neuropsychiatric symptoms in dementia, including those associated with Alzheimer's disease.

Agitation, Wasting, and Other Conditions Associated with Dementia and Alzheimer's Disease

While there is a small possibility that medical cannabis can help with the underlying disease processes in Alzheimer's disease and other types of dementia, the real benefit of medical cannabis in these patients it to treat the underlying symptoms.

As mentioned above, there is evidence that neuropsychiatric symptoms associated with dementia and Alzheimer's disease respond well to medical cannabis. In particular, medical cannabis can be very helpful for agitation. Agitation and anxiety seen with different types of dementia, including Alzheimer's disease, can be mild, in the form of restlessness or pacing, but can also come on suddenly and can be very difficult to manage for caregivers. While common antianxiety or antidepressant prescriptions have been used to treat mild agitation, more severe agitation is often treated by using antipsychotic medications. These medicines can cause serious side effects, including excessive drowsiness, rigidity, and unusual movements. Antipsychotic medications have also been linked to a higher risk of death for patients with dementia, which is why the FDA has placed a "black box" warning on these medications. While all these medications have been used to treat agitation, there is currently no FDA-approved prescription medication indicated for the use of agitation in dementia patients. Medical cannabis, especially low-dose THC, can be calming and help with agitation, without some of the serious adverse effects seen in prescription medications, such as antipsychotics.

In addition to neuropsychiatric symptoms, medical cannabis can help with other symptoms associated with dementia, such as wasting and sleep issues. Wasting or cachexia (the medical term) occurs often because patients with dementia both forget to eat and lose their appetite. Losing weight can predispose them to other medical conditions, and lack of proper nutrition can worsen dementia. The THC found in medical cannabis is known to stimulate appetite and can help with wasting in these patients. Sleep issues are very common in elderly patients in general but can also be particularly problematic in those with dementia. Lack of sleep can also exacerbate the neuropsychiatric symptoms associated with dementia. THC, as well as CBN, are both cannabinoids that are excellent in treating issues related to sleep.

Finally, aging patients in general have several chronic conditions, including chronic pain, which is often from osteoarthritis. Chronic pain can be particularly tricky to manage in patients with dementia and Alzheimer's disease because patients may not be easily able to verbalize their pain symptoms, and patients who are in pain may have increased agitation. There is strong evidence that both CBD and THC found in medical cannabis can help with chronic pain.

Strains for Dementia and Alzheimer's Disease

Cannabis contains many different substances (called cannabinoids) that have medicinal properties. In addition to THC (the component that can make you "high") and CBD (which does not make you high), there are substances called terpenes that give marijuana its smell and flavor. The combination and proportion of cannabinoids and terpenes determine the effects that cannabis has on the body, with different strains of the cannabis plant having different proportions of these substances. The most common way of classifying different strains is dividing them into two categories: indica and sativa. Sativa strains are generally uplifting and energizing, while indica strains are generally more relaxing and sedating. Pinene is a common terpene that is typically found in most sativa strains, and it can be good for memory, as well as a good mood lifter, which is important in patients with dementia and Alzheimer's who tend to have depressed moods when not agitated. Limonene is another good terpene for patients with dementia and Alzheimer's, as it can be calming for patients with agitation. Humulene is a terpene that can decrease appetite, so strains high in humulene should be avoided in patients where wasting is an issue.

There are also hybrid strains, which can be balanced (half indica/half sativa) or more predominant in one or the other. Sativa-predominant hybrid strains can be useful in dementia and Alzheimer's disease when there is need for both uplifting patients while also keeping them calm. While the various strains and terpenes can be effective for dementia, Alzheimer's, and their associated symptoms, every patient is different, so it may take some trial and error to determine which strain is the right strain for your affected loved one. A few strains that patients have successfully used for dementia and Alzheimer's disease include the following:

Sour Diesel and **Green Crack.** Both strains are sativa strains that have a medium (15–20%) amount of THC, with very little (<1%) CBD and are popular for use in patients with dementia and Alzheimer's disease. They appear to be particularly good as mood elevators in these patients who tend to have depressed moods. The both have caryophyllene, which is anti-inflammatory and also helpful with nerve issues. Sour Diesel is also high in limonene, and Green Crack has myrcene, which can also be calming.

Acapulco Gold and **OG Kush** are both sativa-dominant hybrid strains. They are both high in THC (about 15–20%) with very little (less than 1%) CBD. OG Kush is high in myrcene and limonene. Acapulco Gold has caryophyllene as its predominant terpene, as well as myrcene and limonene. Because they are predominantly sativa, they are more uplifting, but as hybrids, they are likely more calming then pure sativa strains.

CBD for Dementia and Alzheimer's Disease

CBD is the nonpsychoactive cannabinoid in medical cannabis and is also found in hemp. It is known to be effective for anxiety, which, as mentioned, is commonly seen in patients with Alzheimer's disease and dementia. However, CBD's effects on Alzheimer's disease and dementia alone are unclear. Unlike anxiety and epilepsy, where there is some research that supports the use of CBD in these conditions, research on cannabis for Alzheimer's disease and dementia (above) is limited, and research on CBD alone is almost nonexistent. CBD has been found in mostly nonhuman studies to be neuroprotective, which means that it has been shown to help lessen the damage of brain cells affected by conditions such as stroke, including the possibility of helping the growth of new brain cells.[7] The mechanism behind CBD's neuroprotective effects are unclear but may be related to reducing inflammation, which can be seen during injury and which is known to sometimes damage healthy tissue. In addition, one study showed that, at least in a test tube, CBD had inhibitory effects on receptors thought to play a role in both Alzheimer's disease (GPR3 receptor) and Parkinson's disease (GPR6 receptor).[8] Whether or not this is applicable to patients with dementia and Alzheimer's disease is still unknown.

However, even without solid evidence that CBD helps patients with Alzheimer's disease and dementia, there are at least two potential benefits for using CBD to treat patients with these conditions. The first is the use of CBD to treat anxiety and agitation, which can be common in all forms of dementia. There is at least some evidence that CBD can help with anxiety in the general population, so this may prove to be helpful in dementia. The second is that CBD appears to counterbalance some of the unwanted effects (sedation, feeling "high") that are associated with THC. While all cannabis strains contain both THC and CBD, many of the strains recommended for Alzheimer's disease and dementia have low levels of CBD. Thus, using CBD combined with high-THC strains that are recommend may be effective in helping with some of these unwanted effects of those strains.

While CBD-only products can be derived from either marijuana or hemp, I generally recommend hemp-derived CBD because it is usually less expensive, and you can obtain this without certification. However, because hemp-derived CBD is not regulated by the FDA, you must be very careful that you are getting a high-quality, full-spectrum, third-party-verified product.

If you decide to try CBD in patients with Alzheimer's disease or other types of dementia, I recommend 25 to 30 mg of CBD a day, which can be ingested by using CBD oil/tincture under the tongue, or CBD oil capsules. CBD, in general, does not immediately alleviate anxiety (or symptoms of Alzheimer's disease and dementia, for that matter), but rather taken daily for at least one to two weeks, it can start to affect some of the chemical signaling in the brain to help alleviate anxiety and possibly help with dementia symptoms. Caregivers should not expect to see improvement in patients' symptoms right away.

Using Different Formulations for Dementia and Alzheimer's Disease

Almost as important as which strain of cannabis you use, or things like the ratio of THC to CBD, is the formulation you use to treat dementia and Alzheimer's disease. Some of this is due to the fact that different formulations have different onsets of actions and different durations. While dementia is always present, certain symptoms like restlessness can be constant and require a long-acting agent, while severe agitation can come on quickly and require a more rapid-acting agent. In addition, patients with dementia may have difficulty with certain formulations, some of which require following a specific set of instructions or commands that must be followed in order to be used correctly.

Pills or capsules (edibles) take longer to work (about an hour hour), but last longer in the body (up to eight hours), so some type of edible is generally preferred for patients with dementia and Alzheimer's disease, both for their long-acting effects and ease of delivery. Depending on the state, some edibles may be available as an indica, sativa, or hybrid and may even be available in a specific strain.

Tinctures are liquids that come in droppers. You place drops of tincture under your tongue to allow for fast absorption, rather than swallowing them directly. Tinctures take about thirty minutes to work and last four to six hours. There are two advantages to tinctures in the treatment of dementia. The first is that they are generally easier to titrate (slowly adjust) the dose, since doses can be increased drop by drop. This is particularly important for elderly patients with dementia, as doses need to be started very low and slowly increased to prevent side effects. Secondly, tinctures may also be easier for caregivers to give patients with dementia, who may not be able to swallow edibles and/ or may not be appropriate for vaping. Finally, while this varies state by state, while most tinctures are extractions of primarily THC and CBD, some tinctures are available in sativa, indica, or hybrid strains, and some states sell extracts of the whole cannabis plant, so you can use a specific strain like the ones listed above.

Vape commonly comes in the form of a concentrated liquid (called "**concentrate**") that is extracted from the cannabis plant, and usually heated so it can be inhaled. Vape also works very quickly (in seconds to minutes), which is very beneficial for acute and severe symptoms. However, it also doesn't last very long (an hour or so), meaning that vape alone is probably not practical for a condition that is always present, like dementia. In addition, vape requires following instructions and some coordination, which may not be possible for certain patients with dementia. Thus, vape may not be the best options for these patients. Where vape may be effective is for acute and severe agitation for patients who are able to follow instructions and coordinate breathing. Almost all cannabis strains come in vape or concentrate, so you can choose one of those listed above (or similar) to start with.

Topical agents can be used to deliver medical cannabis. Salves and creams can be particularly good for aches and pains associated with aging. While topicals aren't going to be used to treat neuropsychiatric symptoms associated with dementia, since chronic pain often occurs in patients with dementia (especially if there is one localized spot), topical agents can be part of a comprehensive cannabis regiment for patients with dementia and Alzheimer's disease.

General Recommendations for Dementia and Alzheimer's Disease

Different people react differently to medications, including medical cannabis. In addition, especially in older patients with dementia, side effects are a concern, so I generally recommend starting with very low doses and slowly increasing the dose to get the desired effect without side effects (dose titration). In addition, since patients with dementia may not be able to verbalize the beneficial effects of cannabis, or any side effects, adjusting the dose may have to rely entirely on caregiver observation. Thus, using medical cannabis in patients with Alzheimer's disease and dementia will require patience.

1. **Start with a high-dose CBD capsule or tincture every day.**
   Since CBD may be neuroprotective, can help with anxiety, and may mitigate some of the side effects of THC, I recommend patients with dementia start with a daily dose of CBD. I recommend 25 mg to 30 mg of CBD a day in a pill/edible/capsule or tincture. This can either be a cannabis-derived CBD or pure-hemp-derived CBD, though I generally recommend hemp-derived CBD, as it is less expensive and easier to obtain, and because there is virtually no THC, it will not make you sleepy or high. Also, since there are no psychoactive effects of CBD alone, there is no need to adjust the dose. You may not see the benefits of CBD for one to two weeks.

2. **Use sativa tinctures or edible two to three times a day.**
   Sativa strains tend to work best in patients with dementia and Alzheimer's disease. They can be uplifting and calming at the same time. Because dementia is something that is always there, edibles can be taken a few times a day to control symptoms all day long. Several companies make edibles that contain 5 mg of THC from a sativa strain that can be helpful for Alzheimer's disease and dementia, and despite having THC, they should not make patients sedated or sleepy. I recommend starting with half a tablet (2.5 mg) two to three times a day and increase by half a tablet each day/dose to determine the amount that helps with several of the associated

symptoms, but does not make patients high. If a patient is not able to take an edible, then tincture would be the next best step. Some edibles also come in dissolvable form and can be placed under the tongue like a tincture. For tinctures, look carefully at the amount of THC per dose. If this is not indicated on the bottle or packing, you may have to figure out the dose yourself. Total milligrams of THC divided by milliliters per bottle is equal to the dose of one dropperful, and there are usually about 20 drops per dropperful. Similar to the edibles, I would start with 2.5 mg of THC per dose. In certain states, it may be possible to get a specific tincture by strain, and I would recommend Sour Diesel or Green Crack.

3. **Address sleep issues by using nighttime cannabis, including indica-based products with potentially higher doses of THC.** Sleep disruption is a commonly associated with dementia, and the lack of a good night's sleep can make the neuropsychiatric symptoms worse. Fortunately, cannabis is also very good at making people sleepy. In addition, to THC and CBD, there is also CBN, which stands for cannabinol. Like CBD, CBN is a nonpsychoactive cannabinoid, and CBN is particularly good for sleep. Five milligrams of CBN may be as effective as a 10-mg dose of diazepam (generic for Valium) for inducing sleep. There are both tinctures and edibles that come in 1:1 CBN:THC ratios. Some also contain natural ingredients such as chamomile and melatonin that can be quite effective to help induce sleep. In addition, some tinctures and edibles contain THC from indica strains, and in some states, you can get tinctures as a whole-plant extract of a particular strain.

Since tinctures only take about twenty to thirty minutes to work, and last about four to six hours, an indica-based tincture, especially one containing CBN, is often a great place to start, as it can help patients both fall asleep and stay asleep. Start with ½ dropperful thirty minutes before bedtime, and increase by a ¼ to ½ dropperful each evening until the patient is falling asleep easily and staying asleep. For patients who have more issues staying asleep than falling asleep, a pill or edible may be a better option. While pills or edibles take about an hour to start working, they last six to eight hours. A 5-mg THC edible, particularly if it is an indica strain and/or contains CBN, would be another good option. Start with a half tablet for the first night or two. If that doesn't work, then go up to one full tablet. You can increase by half a tablet every two nights until the patients is staying asleep.

4. **Use tincture or vape (if possible) on an as-needed basis for acute and severe agitation.**
The combination of daily CBD, daytime sativa, and nighttime indica used in either edible or tincture format should help minimize and acute neuropsychiatric symptoms. However, if they occur, something that works more rapidly make be needed. Vape (also known as concentrate) is also likely the best option for acute episodes of agitation that are common with dementia and Alzheimer's disease. Vape has a very rapid onset of action but may not be possible for a dementia patient to take. If they cannot properly take a vape, a tincture is the next best thing. In some states, you can get strain-specific tinctures that are whole-plant extracts. Thus, sativa hybrids like Acapulco Gold and OG Kush may be helpful. In other states, you may only be able to get a sativa tincture that is not strain specific. However, if more sedation is needed, an indica-leaning hybrid or a pure indica strain may end up working better.

Chapter 19 Notes

1. Hebert, L. E., J. Weuve, P. A. Scherr, and D. A. Evans. Alzheimer disease in the United States (2010-2050) estimated using the 2010 census. *Neurology* 2013 May: 80(19), 1778–83.

2. Terry, R. D., E. Masliah, D. P. Salmon DP, et al. Physical basis of cognitive alterations in Alzheimer's disease: synapse loss is the major correlate of cognitive impairment. *Ann Neurol* 1991 Oct: 30(4), 572–80.

3. Neuropathology Group of the Medical Research Council Cognitive Function and Ageing Study (MRC CFAS). Pathological correlates of late-onset dementia in a multicentre, community-based population in England and Wales. *Lancet* 2001: 357(9251), 169.

4. Cao, C., Y. Li, H. Liu, et al. The Potential Therapeutic Effects of THC on Alzheimer's Disease. *Journal of Alzheimer's Disease* 2014: 42(3), 973–984.

5. Hillen, J. B., N. Soulsby, C. Alderman, and G. E. Caughey. Safety and effectiveness of cannabinoids for the treatment of neuropsychiatric symptoms in dementia: a systematic review. *Therapeutic advances in drug safety* 2019: 10, 1–23.

6. Kwakye, P., and S. McCormack. Medical Cannabis for the Treatment of Dementia: A Review of Clinical Effectiveness and Guidelines-CADTH Rapid Response Report: Summary with Critical Appraisal. *Canadian Agency for Drugs and Technologies in Health* 2019 Jul: 17.

7. Campos, A. C., M. V. Fogaça, A. B. Sonego, and F. S. Guimarães. Cannabidiol, neuroprotection and neuropsychiatric disorders. *Pharmacol Res* 2016 Oct: 112, 119–127.

8. Laun, A. S., and Z. H. Song. GPR3 and GPR6, novel molecular targets for cannabidiol. *Biochemical and Biophysical Research Communications* 2017: 490(1), 17–21.

Chapter 20:

How to Use Medical Cannabis and CBD for Tremor and Parkinson's Disease

What Is Parkinson's Disease?

Parkinson's disease is known as a neurodegenerative disorder, which means there is some destruction of certain nerve cells in the brain, which in turn leads to symptoms. In Parkinson's disease, the nerve cells (called neurons) involved are in the part of the brain called the substantia nigra, and the damaged neurons have problems producing dopamine. Dopamine is a neurotransmitter, which is a chemical substance produced in nerve cells that allows communication between brain cells and other neurons. An abnormal collection of proteins called Lewy bodies can be found in the damaged areas of the substantia nigra. While this is what leads to the symptoms of Parkinson's disease, why it happens or the cause of Parkinson's disease is unknown.

One of the more common symptoms of Parkinson's disease is tremor, which is a shaking of the extremities. Patients with Parkinson's disease also move slowly (called bradykinesia), have stiff moving limbs (rigidity), and have problems with walking and balance. These symptoms generally develop slowly over many years. In addition to tremor and other movement issues (called "motor symptoms"), patients with Parkinson's disease can have a variety of other nonmotor symptoms. Common nonmotor symptoms include depression, lack of interest, constipation, sleep disorders, loss of sense of smell, and cognitive impairment.

While tremor is common is Parkinson's disease, not all tremors are related to Parkinson's. Tremors that happen with rest, or resting tremors, are common in Parkinson's disease as well as other related conditions. However, tremors with movement (kinetic tremors; e.g., trying to write or pick up a glass), are often not related to Parkinson's disease and are usually not even related to any disease. The most common kind of kinetic tremor is called essential tremor and can occur in up to 5% of all adults.[1] These types of tremors are not typically associated with nonmotor symptoms. Even though essential tremors are not serious, they can be bothersome and treated with a variety of therapies, including prescription medications and medical cannabis.

Medical Cannabis for Tremor and Parkinson's Disease

Medical cannabis can be used to treat both essential tremors as well as tremors associated with Parkinson's disease. Medical cannabis can also be used to treat some of the associated symptoms related to Parkinson's disease, especially some of the nonmotor symptoms. Finally, there is a small possibility that medical cannabis could be used to treat the underlying condition causing Parkinson's disease itself.

In terms of treating the underlying condition, there is very limited evidence that cannabis can treat the underlying disease process involved with Parkinson's disease. However, we do know that cannabinoid receptors (CB1) are present in the areas of the brain where dopamine is released. At least in a test tube, studies have shown that blocking CB1 receptors helps make some of the dopamine stimulating drugs used in Parkinson's work better at the dopamine receptor.[2] In addition to CBD, which has been found to have neuroprotective effects, another cannabinoid found in cannabis, Δ9-tetrahydrocannabivarin, or THCV, was, at least in animal research models for Parkinson's disease, found to not only have neuroprotective effects, but also relieve symptoms.[3] However, all this research is far from clear evidence that cannabis can help the underlying process, either in the prevention or treatment of Parkinson's disease.

In relation to tremor, since cannabis (and THC in particular) can be a strong muscle relaxant, one would think that there would be robust evidence for treatment of Parkinson's disease and/or tremor with medical cannabis. Unfortunately, the limited currently available research is not particularly supportive. Several clinical trials were not able to show improvement in motor symptoms in patients with Parkinson's disease. However, there are a few small observational studies that have shown significant improvements in tremor in patients with Parkinson's disease using cannabis, as well as significant improvements in rigidity and bradykinesia.[4] In addition to tremor, some medications used in Parkinson's disease have the side effect of causing involuntary movements or dyskinesias. One very small randomized trial showed that a synthetic cannabinoid receptor blocker could actually decrease dyskinesia when using these prescription medications.[5]

Nonmotor Symptoms Associated with Parkinson's Disease

While there is a small possibility that medical cannabis can help with the underlying disease processes in Parkinson's disease and better evidence that medical cannabis may help with both Parkinsonian and non-Parkinsonian tremors (essential tremors), a major benefit of medical cannabis in patients with Parkinson's disease may be in its ability to help with nonmotor symptoms.

There are many nonmotor symptoms associated with Parkinson's disease. Disorders of mood are common and can include anxiety, depression, apathy, lack of interest, and irritability. Disorders of thought may also occur and include issues with language, memory, and attention; delusions, hallucinations, and even impulse control have all been reported. Related issues that likely involve brain function include problems with sleep. Other nonmotor symptoms include pain, fatigue, constipation, and loss of sense of smell and weight gain/weight loss.[6] There is strong evidence that medical cannabis can help with all of these mood disorders in patients without Parkinson's disease. Medical cannabis can certainly help with sleep and anorexia in patients without

Parkinson's' disease. While there is limited research in the effects of medical cannabis for nonmotor symptoms, there is at least one small study that not only showed improvements in tremor, but also showed significant improvements in nonmotor symptoms such as pain and sleep disorders in patients suffering from Parkinson's disease.[4]

Strains for Tremor and Parkinson's Disease

Cannabis contains many different substances (called cannabinoids) that have medicinal properties. In addition to THC (the component that can make you "high") and CBD (which does not make you high), there are substances called terpenes that give marijuana its smell and flavor. The combination and proportion of cannabinoids and terpenes determine the effects that cannabis has on the body, with different strains of the cannabis plant having different proportions of these substances.

The most common way of classifying different strains is dividing them into two categories: indica and sativa. Sativa strains are generally uplifting and energizing, while indica strains are generally more relaxing and sedating. There are also hybrid strains, which can be balanced (half indica/half sativa) or more predominant in one or the other. Different strains have terpenes that can be effective for patients with tremor and Parkinson's disease. Myrcene is a terpene that is a good muscle relaxant and can be useful in tremor. Limonene is good terpene for patients with Parkinson's disease who get agitated, as it can be calming. Because the strains that are used for motor and nonmotor symptoms may be different, patients with Parkinson's disease may need more than one strain to treat their symptoms. While the various strains and terpenes can be effective for essential and Parkinsonian tremor, as well as some of the nonmotor symptoms associated with Parkinson's disease, every patient is different, so it may take some trial and error to determine which strain is the right one. A few strains that patients have successfully used for Parkinson's disease include the following:

Bubba Kush is a potent indica strain known for its sedative and pain-relieving properties. However, it is also a very good muscle relaxant and thus can be very helpful to relieve spasms and tremor. Bubba Kush has a medium amount (14–19%) of THC, and very little (<1%) CBD. The primary terpenes involved are caryophyllene, which is anti-inflammatory and thus can be helpful with nerve issues, as well as some limonene.

Cherry Cola is an indica-dominant hybrid, containing about 70% indica and 30% sativa. It is higher in THC (21%–25%) and very low (about 1%) in CBD. The primary terpenes involved are beta-myrcene, which relaxes muscles and thus can be good for tremor, as well as limonene. Like Bubba Kush, it has sedative properties and is good for sleep, anxiety, and pain. Not only will it help with muscle spasms and tremor, but it can also help with some of the nonmotor symptoms.

Chem Dawg is a balanced hybrid strain, meaning it has equal amounts of indica and sativa. It is a bit higher (16–22%) in THC and also has very little (<1%) CBD. Its predominant terpenes are caryophyllene, followed by myrcene and a little limonene. This strain may not help so much with tremor but can be effective for some of the nonmotor symptoms related to Parkinson's disease, such as decreased appetite and depression.

Amnesia Haze is a pure sativa strain, meaning that is more uplifting and therefore generally used for conditions such as depression. Like Bubba Kush and Chem Dawg, it has a medium (16–20%) amount of THC, with very little (<1%) CBD. The predominant terpene is myrcene, but this strain is also high in caryophyllene. Because of high amounts of myrcene, it may be effective for tremor without being sedating but can also be useful for some of the nonmotor symptoms related to Parkinson's disease.

CBD for Tremor and Parkinson's Disease

CBD is the nonpsychoactive cannabinoid in medical cannabis and is also found in hemp. It is known to be effective for anxiety, which is commonly seen in patients with Parkinson's disease, and it has anti-inflammatory properties, which may play a role in the halting the progression of Parkinson's disease. However, CBD's effects on tremor and Parkinson's disease alone are unclear. Unlike anxiety and epilepsy, where there is some research that supports the use of CBD in these conditions, research on cannabis for Parkinson's disease (above) is limited, and research on CBD alone is virtually nonexistent. CBD has been found in mostly nonhuman studies to be neuroprotective, which means that it has been shown to help lessen the effects of damaged brain cells in conditions such as stroke, including the possibility of helping the growth of new brain cells.[7] The mechanism behind CBD's neuroprotective effects are unclear but may be related to reducing inflammation, which can be seen during injury and is known to also damage healthy tissue. In addition, one study showed that in a test tube, CBD had inhibitory effects on receptors thought to play a role in both Alzheimer's disease (GPR3 receptor) and Parkinson's disease (GPR6 receptor).[8] Whether or not this is applicable to patients with Parkinson's disease is still unknown.

However, while there may not be strong evidence that CBD helps the underlying condition causing Parkinson's disease, or can effectively treat tremor, CBD may be very effective in treating the nonmotor symptoms associated with Parkinson's disease. CBD can be used to treat anxiety and agitation, which is a common nonmotor symptom seen in Parkinson's disease. There is at least some evidence that CBD can help with anxiety in the general population, and there are at least a few studies where CBD was found to be effective for psychosis and sleep-related disorders when used in patients with Parkinson's disease.[9, 10] Another use for CBD, both in Parkinson's disease and tremor, is that CBD appears to counterbalance some of the unwanted effects (sedation, feeling "high") that is associated with THC. While cannabis strains contain both THC and CBD, many of the strains recommended for Parkinson's disease and tremor have low levels of CBD. Thus, using CBD combined with high-THC strains that are recommend for these patients may be effective in helping with some of the potentially unwanted effects.

While CBD-only products can be derived from either cannabis or hemp, I generally recommend hemp-derived CBD because it is usually less expensive, and you can obtain this without certification. However, because hemp-derived CBD is not regulated by the FDA, you must be very careful that you are getting a high-quality, full-spectrum, third-party-verified product. If you decide to try CBD in patients with Parkinson's disease, I recommend 25 to 30 mg of CBD a day, which can be obtained by using CBD oil/tincture under the tongue, or CBD oil capsules. CBD, in general, does not immediately alleviate anxiety, or symptoms of Parkinson's disease for that matter, but rather, taken daily for at least one to two weeks, it can start to affect some of the chemical signaling in the brain to help alleviate anxiety and possibly help with the progression of Parkinson's disease.

Using Different Formulations for Tremor and Parkinson's Disease

Almost as important as which strain of cannabis you use, or the ratio of THC to CBD, is the formulation used to treat tremor and Parkinson's disease. Some of this is due to the fact that different formulations have different onsets of actions and different durations. While Parkinson's disease is always present, certain symptoms like tremor may be constant and require a longer-acting agent, while a nonmotor symptom like agitation might come on quickly and require a more rapid-acting agent. In addition, patients with Parkinson's, especially with tremor and other motor symptoms, might have difficulty with certain formulations, some of which require finer motor coordination or a steadier hand.

Pills or capsules (edibles) take longer to work (about an hour hour), but last longer in the body (up to eight hours), so edibles are excellent options for tremors as well as nonmotor symptoms that occur most of the time. In addition, edibles are also preferred for the ease of use. Depending on the state, some edibles may be available as an indica, sativa, or hybrid and may even be available in a specific strain.

Tinctures are liquids that come in droppers. You place drops of tincture under your tongue to allow for fast absorption, rather than swallowing them directly. Tinctures take about thirty minutes to work and last four to six hours. There are two advantages to tinctures in the treatment of Parkinson's disease and tremor. The first is that they are generally easier to titrate (slowly adjust) the dose, since doses can be increased drop by drop. This is particularly important for elderly patients, who more commonly have tremor and Parkinson's disease, as doses should be started very low and slowly increased to prevent side effects. Secondly, for patients with Parkinson's disease who have more severe symptoms, tinctures may also be easier for caregivers to give patients who may not be able to swallow edibles and/or may not be appropriate for vaping. Finally, while this varies state by state, while most tinctures are extractions of primarily THC and CBD, some tinctures are available in sativa, indica, or hybrid strains, and some states sell extracts of the whole cannabis plant, so you can use a specific strain, like the ones listed above.

Vape commonly comes in the form of a concentrated liquid (called "**concentrate**") that is extracted from the cannabis plant, and usually heated so it can be inhaled. Vape also works very quickly (seconds to minutes), which is very beneficial for acute and severe symptoms. However, it also doesn't last very long (an hour or so), meaning that vape alone is probably not practical for a condition that can be present continuously, like tremor or some of the nonmotor symptoms of Parkinson's disease. In addition, vape requires following instructions and some coordination, which may not be possible for certain patients with severe tremor or severe nonmotor symptoms from Parkinson's. Thus, vape may not be the best options for all of these patients. Vape may be effective for acute and severe motor or nonmotor symptoms, such as agitation, for patients who are able to follow instructions and coordinate breathing. Almost all cannabis strains come in vape or concentrate, so you can choose one of those listed above (or similar) to start with.

General Recommendations for Tremor and Parkinson's Disease

Different people react differently to medications, including medical cannabis. In addition, especially in older patients, side effects are a concern, so I generally recommend starting with very low doses and slowly increasing the dose to get the desired effect without side effects (dose titration). In addition, patients with Parkinson's disease will likely have both constant symptoms (depressed mood, slow movement) that are there all the time, as well as other symptoms that can come and go (tremor, agitation). This complicates dose adjustments since doses may be different from day to day. Because we want to go "low and slow," while simultaneously needing to change doses based on variable symptoms, using medical cannabis in patients with Parkinson's disease will require patience. In contrast, essential tremor tends to be more regular and is not accompanied by nonmotor symptoms, so use of medical cannabis is a bit simpler (though still will require some patience).

1. **For all patients (Parkinson's disease and other tremors), start with high-dose CBD capsule or tincture every day.**
   Since CBD may be neuroprotective and inhibit certain receptors involved in Parkinson's disease, since it can help mitigate some of the side effects of THC use to treat tremor and nonmotor symptoms, and since CBD alone may be effective for some of the nonmotor symptoms related to Parkinson's disease (anxiety and depression in particular), I recommend that patients with both Parkinson's disease and essential tremor start with a daily dose of CBD. I recommend 25 mg to 30 mg of CBD a day in a pill/edible/capsule or tincture. This can either be a cannabis-derived CBD or pure-hemp-derived CBD, though I generally recommend hemp-derived CBD as it is less expensive and easier to obtain, and because there is virtually no THC, it will not make patients sleepy or high. Also, since there are no psychoactive effects of CBD alone, there is no need to adjust the dose. You may not see the benefits of CBD for one to two weeks.

2. **For tremor, either Parkinsonian or essential tremor, use edible or tincture for continuous tremors, and vape (if possible) for acute worsening of tremors.**
   Both essential tremor and Parkinsonian tremor can be experienced differently by different patients. In general, the tremor is always

there, though under certain circumstances or even certain times of the day, tremor may be worse. Since tremor often occurs throughout the day, an edible or a tincture is preferred. If available, I would recommend an edible or tincture related to a sativa (Amnesia Haze or similar) or balanced hybrid strain (Chem Dawg or similar) to prevent sedation. However, for acute worsening of tremors, or in situations in which tremor is particularly bothersome, vape may be preferred. Vape has a very rapid onset of action but may not be possible for a patient with severe Parkinson's disease to take properly.

3. **For nonmotor Parkinson's symptoms, use sativa tinctures or an edible two to three times a day.**

Sativa strains can be uplifting and calming at the same time. When nonmotor Parkinson symptoms occur, they are often constant, though can occur with episodes of worsening. Therefore, sativa edibles can be taken a few times a day to control symptoms all day long. One advantage of sativa edibles in Parkinson's disease is that the same edible may work for both the motor (see above) and nonmotor symptoms. Several companies make edibles (pills, capsules, gummies) that are 5 mg of THC from a sativa strain, and despite having THC, should not make patients sleepy. I recommend starting with half a tablet (2.5 mg) two to three times a day and increase by half a tablet each day/dose to determine the amount that helps with non-motor symptoms but does not make the patient high. If a patient is not able to take an edible, then tincture would be the next best step. Some edibles also come in dissolvable form and can be placed under the tongue like a tincture. For tinctures, look carefully at the amount of THC per dose. If this is not indicated on the bottle or packing, you may have to figure out the dose yourself. The total milligrams of THC divided by milliliters per bottle is equal to the dose of one dropperful, and there are usually about twenty drops per dropperful. Similar to the edibles, I would start with 2.5 mg of THC per dose. In some states, it is possible to get a strain-specific tincture. If this is the case, I would recommend Amnesia Haze or a strain with a similar cannabinoid and terpene profile.

4. **For Parkinson's disease, address sleep issues by using night-time cannabis, including indica-based products with potentially higher doses of THC.**

Sleep disruption is a common nonmotor symptom of Parkinson's disease, and the lack of a good night's sleep can make both motor and nonmotor symptoms worse. Fortunately, cannabis is also very good at making people sleepy. In addition, to THC and CBD, there is also CBN, which stands for cannabinol. Like CBD, CBN is a nonpsychoactive cannabinoid, and CBN is particularly good for sleep. Five milligrams of CBN may be as effective as a 10-mg dose of diazepam (generic for Valium) for inducing sleep. There are both tinctures and edibles that come in 1:1 CBN:THC ratios. Some also contain natural ingredients such as chamomile and melatonin that can be quite effective to help induce sleep. In addition, some tinctures and edibles contain THC from indica strains, and in some states, you can get tinctures as a whole-plant extract of a particular strain.

Since tinctures only take about twenty to thirty minutes to work, and last about four to six hours, an indica-based tincture, especially one containing CBN, is often a great place to start, as it can help patients both fall asleep and stay asleep. Start with ½ dropperful thirty minutes before bedtime, and increase by a ¼ to ½ dropperful each evening until you are falling asleep easily and staying asleep. For patients who have more issues staying asleep than falling asleep, a pill or edible may be a better option. While pills or edibles take about an hour to start working, they last six to eight hours. A 5-mg THC edible, particularly if it is an indica strain and/or contains CBN, would be another good option. Start with a half tablet for the first night or two. If that doesn't work, then go up to the one full tablet. You can increase by half a tablet every two nights until you are staying asleep.

5. **For acute nonmotor Parkinson's symptoms, such as agitation, use tincture or vape (if possible) on an as-needed basis.**

   The combination of daily CBD, daytime sativa, and nighttime indica used in either edible or tincture format should help minimize tremor as well as nonmotor symptoms in patients with Parkinson's disease. However, if there is an acute worsening of both motor and nonmotor symptoms, something that works more rapidly make be needed. Vape (also known as concentrate) may not only be one of the best options for an acutely worsening or troublesome tremor but can also be a good option for acutely worsening agitation or anxiety. Vape has a very rapid onset of action but may not be possible for a patient with severe Parkinson's disease to take properly. If patients cannot properly take a vape, a tincture is the next best thing. Indicas like Bubba Kush or indica-leaning hybrids sativa hybrids like Acapulco Gold and OG Kush may be helpful. However, if more sedation is needed, indica-leaning hybrids like Cherry Cola may be best for these situations.

Chapter 20 Notes

1. Benito-León, J., F. Bermejo-Pareja, J. M. Morales, et al. Prevalence of essential tremor in three elderly populations of central Spain. *Mov Disord* 2003: 18(4), 389.

2. Rodríguez de Fonseca, F., M. A. Gorriti, A. Bilbao, et al. Role of the endogenous cannabinoid system as a modulator of dopamine transmission: Implications for Parkinson's disease and schizophrenia. *Neurotoxicity Research* 2001: 3:23–35.

3. García, C., C. Palomo-Garo, M. García-Arencibia, et al. Symptom-relieving and neuroprotective effects of the phytocannabinoid Δ9-THCV in animal models of Parkinson's disease. *British Journal of Pharmacology* 2011: 163(7), 1495–1506.

4. Lotan, I., T.A. Treves, Y. Roditi, and R. Djaldetti. Cannabis (medical marijuana) treatment for motor and non-motor symptoms of Parkinson disease: an open-label observational study. *R Clin Neuropharmacol* 2014 Mar–Apr: 37(2), 41–4.

5. Sieradzan, K. A., S. H. Fox, M. Hill, et al. Cannabinoids reduce levodopa-induced dyskinesia in Parkinson's disease: a pilot study. *Neurology* 2001 Dec 11: 57(11), 2108–11.

6. Poewe, W. Non-motor symptoms in Parkinson's disease. *Eur J Neurol* 2008 Apr 15 Suppl: 1, 14–20.

7. Campos, A. C., M. V. Fogaça, A. B. Sonego, and F. S. Guimarães. Cannabidiol, neuroprotection and neuropsychiatric disorders. *Pharmacol Res* 2016 Oct: 112, 119–127.

8. Laun, A. S., and Z. H. Song. GPR3 and GPR6, novel molecular targets for cannabidiol. *Biochemical and Biophysical Research Communications*, 2017: 490(1), 17–21.

9. Zuardi, A. W., J. A. Crippa, J. E. Hallak, et al. Cannabidiol for the treatment of psychosis in Parkinson's disease. *Psychopharmacol* 2009 Nov: 23(8), 979–83.

10. Chagas, M. H., A. L. Eckeli, A. W. Zuardi, et al. Cannabidiol can improve complex sleep-related behaviours associated with rapid eye movement sleep behaviour disorder in Parkinson's disease patients: a case series. *J Clin Pharm Ther* 2014 Oct: 39(5), 564–6.

Chapter 21:

How to Use Medical Cannabis and CBD for Autism

What Is Autism?

Autism is a complex neurobehavioral disorder that usually appears before the age of three, where problems with the brain lead to issues with normal development. Developmental issues cause autistic children to have problems with social interaction, communication, and thought processes.[1] Autism was once thought to be rare, but now current estimates are that one in every fifty-nine children may have autism or be on the autism spectrum.[2] Autism is characterized by impairment in reciprocal social interaction, impairment in communication, and the presence of repetitive patterns of movement, behaviors, interests, and activities.[3] Repetitive behaviors include complex rituals and unusual movements such as rocking and hand flapping. In addition to issues related to problems with development, children with autism also frequently suffer from other seemingly unrelated conditions, such as allergies, asthma, epilepsy, digestive disorders, sleeping disorders, and others. There is currently no cure for autism, though early behavioral interventions and treatments may help. However, pharmaceutical approaches are currently used to manage some of the more serious and bothersome symptoms. Antipsychotic medicines such as risperidone (Risperdal) and aripiprazole (Abilify) are used to treat irritability and aggression, stimulants like methylphenidate (Ritalin) are used to treat hyperactivity and inattention, antidepressants like fluoxetine (Prozac) are used to treat repetitive behaviors, and sleeping aids like mirtazapine

(Remeron) are used for insomnia. Unfortunately, many of these medications have unwanted side effects, to which children are particularly sensitive.[4]

Medical Cannabis for Autism

While there is limited scientific evidence supporting the use of medical cannabis and CBD in the treatment of autism, it is currently a qualifying condition in five states (Delaware, Pennsylvania, Minnesota, Georgia, and South Carolina). Thus, there is at least enough anecdotal evidence and some research that advocates in those states were able to get the condition listed.

Animal studies suggest that cannabinoids may play a role in treating some of the deficits seen in autism. Mice can be bred to have a form of mental retardation called fragile X mental retardation (FMR1) that also show some of the core symptoms of autism spectrum disorder (ASD) including deficits in social interactions, repetitive behaviors, and hyperactivity. Several studies have identified alterations in the endocannabinoid system, which may be linked to the ASD-like symptoms displayed in the FMR1 mice.[5, 6] Cannabidivarin, or CBDV, is a less common cannabinoid that can alter electrical activity in brain, including reducing spikes associated with disruptive and aggressive behavior. In one study of rats developing ASD-like symptoms from prenatal exposure to valproic acid, subjects receiving CBDV showed improvements in social behavior and repetitive movements.[7] Oxytocin has also been used to treat ASD,[4] due to its role in the regulation of social reward. Researchers have shown that problems with oxytocin-driven anandamide signaling (anandamide being one of the primary endocannabinoids) may be defective in ASD, and that correcting these deficits might offer a strategy to treat ASD.[8] Finally, there is evidence that CBD effects neurotransmitters, including glutamate-GABA systems, that may be altered in ASD, and thus CBD may have a role.[9]

In terms of research treating of actual patients with autism, there is some data supporting the use of medical cannabis seen in three studies done in Israel. In one Israeli study of 155 patients using a cannabis oil low in THC (1.5% THC and 30% CBD), researchers found that of the 93 parents who responded to interviews after six months of treatment, 28 patients (30.1%) reported a significant improvement, 50 (53.7%) moderate, 6 (6.4%) slight, and 8 (8.6%) had no change in their condition.[10] Another Israeli study using cannabidiol in 53 children for over two months found self-injury and rage attacks improved in 34 patients (67.6%), hyperactivity symptoms improved in 28 patients (68.4%), and sleep issues improved in 21 patients (71.4%).[11] The third retrospective study followed 60 children who had ASD with severe behavioral issues and were given CBD and THC in a 20:1 ratio, derived from whole-plant extract dissolved in olive oil. Following the cannabis treatment, behavioral outbreaks were much improved or very much improved in 61% of patients. Similar to the other studies, adverse events were minimal and included sleep disturbances (14%), irritability (9%), and loss of appetite (9%).[12] Thus, clinical evidence does support the use of medical cannabis in autism and ASD.

In addition to efficacy and safety, there are several other issues to consider when using medical cannabis and CBD for the treatment of autism and ASD. First, while THC likely has a low risk of side effects, especially when using in the low doses typical of medical cannabis treatment, there is animal research and some human research that shows early exposure to marijuana can have negative impacts on the brain in terms of learning and memory. Thus, use of medical cannabis in children must be done very cautiously.[13] In addition, children are minors and thus cannot get medical cannabis by themselves, and in younger children, it needs to be administered by a caregiver, so certain formulations like vape may not be appropriate.

Treating Agitation, Repetitive Behaviors, Hyperactivity, Seizures and Insomnia in Autism

While there is some evidence to suggest that medical cannabis can help with some of the underlying disease processes that causes autism and ASD, the real benefit of medical cannabis in these patients is to treat the associated symptoms. While behavioral approaches have been effective, in many cases prescriptions medications are also used, most of which have undesired side effects. The previously discussed research suggests that medical cannabis and CBD can be effectively used to treat the symptoms of autism and ASD, while possibly helping the underlying disease process, without the unwanted side effects seen in prescription use.

One of the most bothersome symptoms of autism and ASD as described by caregivers is agitation. Medical cannabis can be very helpful for agitation. Agitation is commonly seen with autism, often in the form of irritability and aggression. Agitation can come on suddenly and can be exceedingly difficult to manage for parents and other caregivers. It is not uncommon to manage agitation using antipsychotic medications like risperidone (Risperdal). These medicines can cause serious side effects, including excessive drowsiness, rigidity, and unusual movements. Repetitive behaviors can occur frequently throughout the day or occur suddenly, as seen in agitation. Pharmaceuticals such as antidepressants have been used for this, but cannabis and CBD may be a safer alternative. Hyperactivity is also frequently associated in patients with autism and ASD. While there are no specific studies looking at cannabis and this particular condition, there is certainly a role for medical cannabis in the treatment of patients with ADHD who do not have autism, as discussed in Chapter 16. Similarly, seizures are another common condition in patients with autism and ASD, and there is an abundance of evidence for using medical cannabis and CBD in the treatment of seizures. In fact, Epidiolex is a cannabis-derived FDA-approved prescription medication for the treatment of certain types of seizures seen in children. Finally, sleep disorders are also seen in autism, and medical cannabis is excellent for helping with sleep. Lack of sleep can also exacerbate agitation and other symptoms associated with autism and ASD. THC, as well as CBN, are both cannabinoids that are excellent in treating issues related to sleep.

Strains for Autism

Cannabis contains many different substances (called cannabinoids) that have medicinal properties. In addition to THC (the component that can make you "high") and CBD (which does not make you high), there are substances called terpenes that give marijuana its smell and flavor. The combination and proportion of cannabinoids and terpenes determine the effects that cannabis has on the body, with different strains of the cannabis plant having different proportions of these substances leading to different effects. The most common way of classifying different strains is dividing them into two categories: indica and sativa. Sativa strains are generally uplifting and energizing, while indica strains are generally more relaxing and sedating. Limonene is an excellent terpene for patients with autism, as it can be calming for patients with agitation. Linalool and myrcene are two additional terpenes that can be calming.

In addition to indica and sativa, there are also hybrid strains, which can be balanced (half indica/half sativa) or more predominant in one or the other. Certain sativa and sativa-predominant-hybrid strains tend to be preferred in autistic children because they tend to be less sedating. However, certain indica-leaning strains can be particularly useful for sleep and acute agitation. While the various strains and terpenes can be effective for autism and ASD, every patient is different, so it may take some trial and error to determine which strain is the right strain for each patient. A few strains that patients have successfully used for autism and ASD include the following:

Sour Diesel and **Green Crack.** These are both sativa strains that have a medium (15–20%) amount of THC, with very little (<1%) CBD and are popular for use in patients with autism. Sour Diesel is also high in limonene, and Green Crack has myrcene, both of which can also be calming.

Blue Dream is a sativa-predominant hybrid strain that also has a medium (16–20%) amount of THC, with very little (<1%) CBD. It has myrcene as its predominant terpene, which can help with relaxation.

Northern Lights is a pure indica with a medium (14–19%) amount of THC, and very little (<1%) CBD. Its predominant terpenes are myrcene and caryophyllene. It is useful for insomnia and agitation.

Hindu Kush is also a pure indica strain named after a mountain range between Pakistan and Afghanistan, where it originated. Hindu Kush has a medium (15–19%) amount of THC, with very little (<1%) CBD. Its main terpene is limonene, which is also calming. Thus, this strain is also good for sleep and agitation.

CBD for Autism

CBD is the nonpsychoactive cannabinoid in medical cannabis and is also found in hemp. It is known to be effective for anxiety and seizures, which can sometimes be seen in autism and ASD and substantially impact the quality of life for these individuals. Thus, CBD provides a viable treatment option for the multiple neurological pathologies seen in autism and ASD.[14] The mechanism of the benefit for CBD in autism and ASD is not entirely clear. We know that CBD has been found in mostly nonhuman studies to be neuroprotective, which means that it has been shown to help lessen the damage of brain cells affected by conditions such as stroke, including the possibility of helping the growth of new brain cells,[15] so this might play a role. As mentioned, some of CBD's benefit may be acting on certain neurotransmitters.[9] In fact, in the three Israeli trials showing clinical benefit in patients, all had very high amounts of CBD compared to THC. [10, 11, 12]

In addition to this evidence that CBD can help patients with autism and ASD, another reason to consider using CBD in patients with these conditions is that CBD appears to counterbalance some of the unwanted effects (sedation, feeling "high") that are associated with THC. While all cannabis strains contain both THC and CBD, many of the strains recommended for autism have low levels of CBD. Thus, using CBD combined with high-THC strains that are recommend may be effective in helping with some of these unwanted effects of those strains.

While CBD-only products can be derived from either marijuana or hemp, I generally recommend hemp-derived CBD because it is usually less expensive, and you can obtain this without certification. However, because hemp-derived CBD is not regulated by the FDA, you must be very careful that you are getting a high-quality, full-spectrum, third-party-verified product.

If you decide to try CBD in patients with autism and ASD, I recommend 25 to 30 mg of CBD a day, which can be ingested by using CBD oil/tincture under the tongue, or CBD oil capsules. CBD, in general, does not immediately alleviate agitation, anxiety, or other symptoms related to autism, but rather, taken daily for at least one to two weeks, it can start to affect some of the chemical signaling in the brain to help alleviate agitation, anxiety, seizures, and other associated symptoms. Parents and other caregivers should not expect to see improvement in patients' symptoms right away.

Using Different Formulations for Autism

Almost as important as which strain of cannabis you use, or things like the ratio of THC to CBD, is the formulation you use to treat autism and ASD. Some of this is due to the fact that different formulations have different onsets of actions and different durations. While autism is always present, certain symptoms like irritability and restlessness can be constant and require a long-acting agent, while severe agitation can come on quickly and require a more rapid-acting agent. In addition, patients with autism and ASD are generally children, who develop symptoms as early as three years old. Thus, certain formulations, particularly vape, while effective, may not be perceived as appropriate for children to use. Also, children with autism and ASD can be particularly sensitive to taste, so certain liquids that may be appropriate and excellent to use may not be agreeable to patients based on characteristics of taste due to terpenes involved.

Pills or capsules (edibles) take longer to work (about an hour hour), but last longer in the body (up to eight hours), so some type of edible is generally preferred for patients with autism and ASD both for their long-acting effects and ease of delivery. In addition, some edibles come in the form of pleasant-tasting gummies, candy, and even chocolate, making adherence to medication much easier. While most edibles do take a long time to work, there are some states that make sublingual tablets that have a more rapid onset of action. Depending on the state, some edibles may be available as an indica, sativa, or hybrid and may even be available in a specific strain.

Tinctures are liquids that come in droppers. You place drops of tincture under your tongue to allow for fast absorption, rather than swallowing them directly. Tinctures take about thirty minutes to work and last four to six hours. There are two advantages to using tinctures in patients with autism. The first is that they are generally easier to titrate (slowly adjust) the dose, since doses can be increased drop by drop. This is particularly important for children, as doses need to be started very low and slowly increased to prevent side effects. Secondly, tinctures may also be easier for parents and caregivers to give patients with autism and ASD who may not be able to swallow certain edibles and/or may not be appropriate for vaping. Finally, while this varies state by state, while most tinctures are extractions of primarily THC and CBD, some tinctures are available in sativa, indica, or hybrid strains, and some states sell extracts of the whole cannabis plant, so you can use a specific strain, like the ones listed above. These whole-plant tinctures are more likely to have a more unpleasant taste, so this needs to be kept in mind in autistic children who are taste-sensitive.

Vape commonly comes in the form of a concentrated liquid (called "**concentrate**") that is extracted from the cannabis plant, and usually heated so it can be inhaled. Vape also works very quickly (in seconds to minutes), which is greatly beneficial for acute and severe symptoms. However, it also doesn't last very long (an hour or so), meaning that vape alone is probably not practical for a condition that is always present, like autism. In addition, vape requires following instructions and some coordination, which may not be possible for certain patients with autism, and parents might not think it appropriate for using a formulation that appears to be like smoking. Thus, vape may not be the best options for these patients. However, vape is highly effective for acute and severe agitation, which tends to be one of the biggest challenges for parents and caregivers. Thus, risks and benefits should be appropriately considered. Almost all cannabis strains come in vape or concentrate, so you can choose one of those listed above (or similar) to start with.

General Recommendations for Autism

Different people react differently to medications, including medical cannabis. In addition, especially in children with autism in whom side effects are a concern, I generally recommend starting with very low doses and slowly increasing the dose to get the desired effect without side effects (dose titration). In addition, since patients with autism and ASD are usually not be able to verbalize the beneficial effects of cannabis or side effects, adjusting the dose usually needs to rely entirely on parent or caregiver observation. Thus, using medical cannabis in patients with autism or ASD will require a lot of patience.

1. **Start with a high-dose CBD edible or tincture every day for general improvement.**
   Since CBD may be neuroprotective, can help with certain symptoms on its own (anxiety, agitation, seizures) and may mitigate some of the side effects of THC, I recommend patients with autism start with a daily dose of CBD. I recommend 25 to 30 mg of CBD a day in a pill/edible/capsule or tincture. This can either be a cannabis-derived CBD or pure-hemp-derived CBD, though I generally recommend hemp-derived CBD as it is less expensive and easier to obtain, and because there is virtually no THC, it will not make children sleepy or high. Also, since there are no psychoactive effects of CBD alone, there is no need to adjust the dose. You may not see the benefits of CBD for one to two weeks. Note that many of the whole-plant CBD tinctures have a strong taste, which may be an issue for children with autism and ASD.

2. **Address sleep issues by using nighttime cannabis, including indica-based products, with cautious use of THC and CBN.**
Sleep disruption is a commonly associated with autism, and the lack of a good night's sleep can make the many of the associated symptoms worse. Fortunately, cannabis is also very good at making people sleepy. In addition, to THC and CBD, there is also CBN, which stands for cannabinol. Like CBD, CBN is a nonpsychoactive cannabinoid, and CBN is particularly good for sleep. Five milligrams of CBN may be as effective as a 10-mg dose of diazepam (generic for Valium) for inducing sleep. There are both tinctures and edibles that come in 1:1 CBN:THC ratios. Some also contain natural ingredients such as chamomile and melatonin that can be quite effective to help induce sleep. In addition, some tinctures and edibles contain THC from indica strains, and in some states, you can get tinctures as a whole-plant extract of a particular strain.

Since tinctures only take about twenty to thirty minutes to work and last about four to six hours, an indica-based tincture, especially one containing CBN, is often a great place to start as it can help patients both fall asleep and stay asleep. Start with ½ a dropperful thirty minutes before bedtime, and increase by a ¼ to ½ dropperful each evening until the patient is falling asleep easily and staying asleep. For children who have more issues staying asleep than falling asleep, or for those who have a hard time using tinctures, a pill or edible may be a better option. While pills or edibles take about an hour to start working, they last six to eight hours. A 5-mg THC edible, particularly if it is an indica strain and/or contains CBN, would be another good option. Start with a half tablet for the first night or two. If that doesn't work, then go up to the one full tablet. You can increase by half a tablet every two nights until the patient is staying asleep.

3. **Consider using sativa tinctures or edibles two to three times a day to minimize regular symptoms.**
Sativa strains tend to work well in children with autism and ASD. They can be calming, without being sedating, and while stimulating

(similar to stimulant prescriptions), they tend to have the opposite effects on hyperactivity and inattention. Because these symptoms of autism are usually always present, edibles can be taken a few times a day to control symptoms all day long. Several companies make edibles that contain 5 mg of THC from a sativa strain that can be helpful for autism and, despite having THC, should not make patients sedated or sleepy. I recommend starting with half a tablet (2.5 mg) two to three times a day and increase by half a tablet each day/dose to determine the amount that helps with several of the associated symptoms, but does not make patients high. If a child is not able to take an edible, then tincture would be the next best step. Some edibles also come in dissolvable form and can be placed under the tongue like a tincture. For tinctures, look carefully at the amount of THC per dose. If this is not indicated on the bottle or packing, you may have to figure out the dose yourself. Total milligrams of THC divided by milliliters per bottle is equal to the dose of one dropperful, and there are usually about 20 drops per dropperful. Like the edibles, I would start with 2.5 mg of THC per dose. In certain states, it may be possible to get a specific tincture by strain, and I would recommend Blue Dream, Sour Diesel, or Green Crack.

4. **Use tincture, fast-acting edibles, or vape (if possible) on an as-needed basis for acute and severe agitation.**
   The combination of daily CBD, daytime sativa, and nighttime indica used in either edible or tincture should help with many of the symptoms associated with autism and ASD. However, certain symptoms, especially agitation, can come on acutely and may be severe, and if that occurs, something that works more rapidly may be needed. Vape (also known as concentrate) is likely the best option for acute episodes of agitation. Vape has a very rapid onset of action but may not be possible for a patient with autism to take and/or parents may not feel comfortable with children using this type of device. Vape is generally available in multiple strains, and thus for acute use in autism, I would recommend Northern Lights or Hindu

Kush. If patients cannot use a vape, a tincture is the next best thing. In some states, you can get strain-specific tinctures that are whole-plant extracts. Again, indicas like Northern Lights or Hindu Kush are recommended for acute use. In other states, you may only be able to get an indica tincture that is not strain specific.

Chapter 21 Notes

1. National Autism Association. https://nationalautismassociation.org/resources/autism-fact-sheet. Accessed 5/2/2020.

2. Centers for Disease Control and Prevention. Data and statistics autism spectrum disorder (ASD): Centers for disease control and prevention; 2018. https://www.cdc.gov/ncbddd/autism/data.html.

3. Association for Science in Treatment of Autism. https://asatonline.org/for-parents/what-is-autism. Accessed 5/2/2020.

4. LeClerc, S., and D. Easley. Pharmacological Therapies for Autism Spectrum Disorder: A Review. *P T* 2015 Jun: 40(6), 389–397.

5. Zhang, L., and B. E. Alger. Enhanced endocannabinoid signaling elevates neuronal excitability in fragile X syndrome. *J Neurosci* 2010: 30, 5724–9.

6. Maccarrone, M., S. Rossi, M. Bari, et al. Abnormal mGlu 5 receptor/endocannabinoid coupling in mice lacking FMRP and BC1 RNA. *Neuropsychopharmacol* 2010: 35, 1500–9.

7. Zamberletti, E., M. Gabaglio, M. Woolley-Roberts, et al. Cannabidivarin Treatment Ameliorates Autism Like Behaviors and Restores Hippocampal Endocannabinoid System and Glia Alterations Induced by Prenatal Valproic Acid Exposure in Rats. *Front Cell Neurosci* 2019: 13, 367.

8. Wei, D., D. Lee, C. D. Cox, et al. Endocannabinoid signaling mediates oxytocin-driven social reward. *PNAS* November 10, 2015: 112(45), 14084–14089.

9. Busquets-Garcia, A., M. Gomis-González, T. Guegan, et al. Targeting the endocannabinoid system in the treatment of fragile X syndrome. *Nat Med* 2013: 19, 603–7.

10. Bar-Lev Schleider, L., R. Mechoulam, N. Saban, G. Meiri, and V. Novack. Real life experience of medical cannabis treatment in autism: analysis of safety and efficacy. *Sci Rep* 2019: 9, 200.

11. Barchel, D., O. Stolar, T. De-Haan, T. Ziv-Baran, N. Saban, D. O. Fuchs, et al. Oral cannabidiol use in children with autism spectrum disorder to treat related symptoms and co-morbidities. *Front Pharmacol* 2019: 9.

12. Aran, A., H. Cassuto, A. Lubotzky, N. Wattad, and E. Hazan. Brief report: Cannabidiol-rich cannabis in children with autism Spectrum disorder and severe behavioral problems—a retrospective feasibility study. *J Autism Dev Disord* 2018.

13. National Institute on Drug Abuse. What are marijuana's long-term effects on the brain? https://www.drugabuse.gov/publications/research-reports/marijuana/what-are-marijuanas-long-term-effects-brain. Accessed 5/2/2020.

14. Gu B. Cannabidiol provides viable treatment opportunity for. *Glob Drugs Ther* 2017: 2, 1–4.

15. Campos, A. C., M. V. Fogaça, A. B. Sonego, and F. S. Guimarães. Cannabidiol, neuroprotection and neuropsychiatric disorders. *Pharmacol Res* 2016 Oct: 112, 119–127.

Chapter 22:

How to Use Medical Cannabis and CBD for Irritable Bowel Syndrome, Crohn's Disease, and Ulcerative Colitis

What Is Irritable Bowel Syndrome?

To start with, in medical terms, a syndrome is constellation of symptoms that occur together where the cause is unclear. Once the cause is known, this becomes a disease. Down syndrome, for example, got its name from an English physician, Dr. John Langdon Down, who in 1862 first noticed similarities in children born with intellectual delays and certain physical features such as a flattened face, a short neck, and small ears. Science would eventually discover that this syndrome was caused by a genetic abnormality in which affected individuals have an extra copy (there are normally two) of the chromosome 21. The medical term for this condition is Trisomy 21, though the term *Down syndrome* is still in use today.

Irritable bowel syndrome, or IBS, is one of the most common gastrointestinal disorders in the United States, with more than 10% of people affected.[1] Affected patients have abdominal pain, which is associated with distention, bloating, and cramping usually occurring with constipation, diarrhea, or both.[2] There are no clinical tests for IBS, and therefore the diagnosis of IBS is made clinically, meaning if you have certain symptoms that fit these patterns and there is no other obvious cause, you will be diagnosed with IBS. As with other syndromes, the causes of IBS remain unclear. While it can be associated with stress and anxiety, some research indicates that a disturbance in the balance of healthy and unhealthy bacteria in the gut may play a role.[3] Other research points to a disorder of brain-gut function, potentially involving neurotransmitters.[4] (Neurotransmitters are the chemical messengers in our body that relay messages from one nerve cell or neuron to another.) Treatment usually consists of dietary modifications (going gluten free or lactose free), medications that treat the symptoms (antidiarrheal agents, laxatives), and a few prescription medications that attempt to get at some of the causes of IBS, including probiotics and antibiotics, as well as medications that work on neurotransmitters.[5]

Since the cause is unclear, and especially given its association with stress, depression, and anxiety, there are some physicians that believe IBS is entirely psychosomatic. This can leave patients feeling very frustrated, with the impression that they are not being heard or believed, or that their medical illness is somehow their fault. However, IBS is a very real and often debilitating condition, even if the cause isn't entirely clear. Fortunately, because medical cannabis and CBD work on a variety of areas that are believed to have an important role in IBS, such as anxiety and neurotransmitters, it can be quite an effective treatment for many patients.

What Is Inflammatory Bowel Disease?

Unlike IBS, which is a syndrome, inflammatory bowel disease, or IBD, is a disease because the causes are known. The two main types of IBD are Crohn's disease and ulcerative colitis. There cause is felt to be a problem with immune system, where the body perceives food or other substances in the digestive tract as a foreign invader (like an infection or cancer) and mounts an immune response leading to inflammation.[6] This chronic inflammation leads to damage of the intestinal tissues, which in turn lead to symptoms including abdominal pain, diarrhea, weight loss, and malnutrition. There are several differences between the two entities; the main difference is that Crohn's disease can occur anywhere in the digestive tract (mouth to anus), and ulcerative colitis is limited to the colon. Since the disease is caused by inflammation and the immune system, most treatments focus on decreasing inflammation and managing symptoms. While there have been recent breakthroughs in medications to treat these conditions, these medications don't resolve all symptoms in all patients. Thus, medical cannabis and CBD may have an important role in treatment for some patients suffering from IBD.

Medical Cannabis and CBD for Irritable Bowel Syndrome and Inflammatory Bowel Disease

As mentioned, the cause of IBS is unknown, but research into potential causes suggests a role for medical cannabis and CBD as potentially effective treatments. While there are no human clinical trials of medical cannabis and CBD being used to treat IBS, there is some research that clarifies this role. First, in addition to migraines, both fibromyalgia (another pain-related syndrome) and IBS are thought to all have a commonality in that patients with these conditions have low levels or a deficiency of their own natural cannabinoids (endocannabinoids).[7] Thus, supplementation of low levels of endocannabinoids by plant based cannabinoids (phytocannabinoids) makes logical sense and is essentially treating the disease and not just the symptoms. Studies have even shown that cannabinoids can block some of the mechanisms that promote pain in headache, fibromyalgia, and IBS.[7]

In terms of IBD, medical cannabis and CBD can treat both pain and inflammation. Studies have shown that changes in endocannabinoid system play an important role in the development of IBD, and there are even studies in mice showing benefits in using cannabis to treat colitis.[8] THC, the psychoactive component in cannabis, binds to CB receptors in the intestinal tract, and CBD can increase levels of anandamide, both leading to reduced inflammation.[8] In fact, in at least one small study of thirteen patients suffering from IBD for many years, three months of treatment with inhaled cannabis was shown to improve their quality of life, reduce their disease activity, and lead to weight gain.[9]

Strains for Irritable Bowel Syndrome, Crohn's Disease, and Ulcerative Colitis

The cannabis plant contains many different substances (called cannabinoids) that have medicinal properties. In addition to THC (the component that can make you "high") and CBD (which does not make you high), there are substances called terpenes that give cannabis its smell and flavor. The combination and proportion of cannabinoids and terpenes will help determine which strains are best to treat your specific medical condition. Beta-caryophyllene is a terpene that has a black pepper taste and smell and is helpful for both pain and inflammation. Myrcene is another terpene that can also be found in hops, mango, and lemongrass, and has muscle-relaxation properties in addition to helping with pain. Terpinolene has a floral aroma and can be found in apples, lilacs, and nutmeg; it is commonly used in soaps and perfumes and known to be sedating. Strains can be indicas, which tend to be more sedating, sativas, which tend to be more uplifting, or hybrids of the two types. While every patient is different, patients with IBS and IBD tend to do better with sativa or hybrid strains. While different strains can be effective for IBS and IBD, every patient is different, so it may take some trial and error to determine which strain is the right strain for you. A few strains that patients have successfully used for IBS and IBD include the following:

Durban Poison is a pure sativa strain that is often associated with treating conditions such as anxiety, depression, and stress. It contains a medium (14–19%) amount of THC, with very little (<1%) CBD. Its predominant terpene is terpinolene followed by myrcene.

Harlequin is a sativa-dominant hybrid with a higher CBD-to-THC ratio (5:2, with about 4–7% THC and 8–16% CBD). It is high in myrcene and can be effective for abdominal pain without causing sedation and can actually be energizing. Thus, it is a popular daytime option.

Blue Dream is a sativa-predominant hybrid strain that has a medium (16–20%) amount of THC, with very little (<1%) CBD. Its predominant terpene is myrcene.

White Widow is a balanced hybrid strain which has about 20% THC and 1% CBD that works well for all types of pain and can improved mood and cause relaxation.

Cannatonic is a balanced hybrid, but like Harlequin, has low amounts (3–7%) of THC, and medium amounts (6–10%) of CBD, with myrcene as a predominant terpene.

CBD for Irritable Bowel Syndrome, Crohn's Disease, and Ulcerative Colitis

While THC, the psychoactive component of medical cannabis, is extremely effective for pain associated with IBS and IBD, CBD may also be useful in these conditions, primarily for its antianxiety and anti-inflammatory properties. Inflammation play a key role in IBD (Crohn's and ulcerative colitis) and may play a role in IBS. IBS is associated with stress and anxiety, and CBD has been found to be effective at treating anxiety. While there are a few small studies that show high-dose CBD might reduce acute anxiety before a stressful event, such as public speaking,[10] CBD has better evidence if taken on a daily basis at lower doses (around 25 mg daily) to reduce general anxiety.[11] The mechanism for CBD's effect on anxiety appears to be on modulation of neurotransmitters. These same neurotransmitters exist in the gastrointestinal tract, and thus CBD may play a role in mitigating the pain response. In fact, neurotransmitter modulations such antidepressant medications are commonly used to treat IBS.[5] IBD is a disease of chronic inflammation, and CBD has known anti-inflammatory effects. While there are no known studies of using CBD alone to treat IBD, CBD may have direct effects on inflammatory cells,[12] and at least in experimental model using rats, CBD was able to prevent pain caused by joint inflammation.[13] Interestingly, IBD is also associated with joint inflammation.

CBD can be taken alone or combined with a very low dose of THC and be quite effective for managing stomach issues, especially during the day. Even though THC has some psychoactive properties, a very low dose of THC should not make you "high" or sleepy. While you can use both cannabis-derived CBD, or hemp-derived CBD for daily use for treating symptoms related to IBS and IBD, I recommend hemp-derived CBD because it is generally less expensive and you can obtain this without certification. However, because hemp-derived CBD is not regulated by the FDA, you must be very careful that you are getting a high-quality, full-spectrum, third-party-verified product. For patients with IBS and IBD, I recommend 25 to 30mg of CBD a day, which can be taken by using CBD oil/tincture under the tongue, or CBD oil capsules.

Using Different Formulations for Irritable Bowel Syndrome, Crohn's Disease, and Ulcerative Colitis

Almost as important as which strain of cannabis you use, or the ratio of THC to CBD, is the formulation you use to treat IBS and IBD. This is because different formulations have different onsets of actions and different durations. Acute or severe pain, which can occur with both IBS and IBD, requires a rapid onset of action (works in seconds or minutes), while Crohn's and ulcerative colitis, being diseases of chronic inflammation, may do better with agents that are taken daily to last a long time.

Tinctures are liquids that come in droppers. You drop tinctures under your tongue to allow for fast absorption rather than swallowing them directly. Tinctures take about thirty minutes to work and last four to six hours, so they can be excellent for regular chronic symptoms related to IBS and IBD. Tinctures are also slightly easier to titrate (adjust the dose), as they can be increased drop by drop. Finally, while this varies state by state, while most tinctures are extractions of primarily THC and CBD, some tinctures are available in sativa, indica, or hybrid strains, and some states sell extracts of the whole cannabis plant, so you can use a specific strain, like the ones listed above.

Pills or capsules (edibles) take a bit longer to work (one to two hours), but last longer in the body (up to eight hours), so they can be an excellent choice for constant pain, or prevention of recurring pain due to inflammation. Depending on the state, some edibles may be available as an indica, sativa, or hybrid and may even be available in a specific strain.

Vape comes in the form of a concentrated liquid (called "**concentrate**") that is extracted from the cannabis plant, and usually heated so it can be inhaled. Vape also works very quickly (in seconds to minutes), which is very beneficial for acute and severe pain, including cramps that can result from either IBS or IBD. However, vape doesn't last very long (an hour or so), meaning that any sedation or other effects will disappear quickly, so you can get back to your day. Almost all cannabis strains come in vape or concentrate, so you can choose one of those listed above (or similar) to start with.

General Recommendations for Irritable Bowel Syndrome, Crohn's Disease, and Ulcerative Colitis

While IBS and IBD are different in both their causes and how patients are affected, the approach to using medical cannabis and CBD for each is not all that different, though the relative importance of the different components of the following regimen may vary, depending on how a patient individually experiences their symptoms.

1. **Treat irritable bowel syndrome, Crohn's disease, and ulcerative colitis by taking a high-dose CBD capsule pill or tincture (with or without small dose of THC) every day.**

    While the role for CBD in IBS may be more about neurotransmitters, and the role for CBD in Crohn's or ulcerative colitis have more to do with inflammation, given that CBD can help with both, I recommend that any patient with IBS or IBD take CBD daily. While CBD will not relieve acute pain, it should generally help the overall condition, reducing symptoms long term, in more of preventative manner. Start with 25 mg to 30 mg of CBD a day in a pill/edible/capsule or tincture. This can either be a cannabis-derived

CBD or a pure-hemp-derived CBD. I generally recommend hemp-derived CBD, as it is less expensive and easier to obtain, and because there is virtually no THC, it will not make you sleepy or high.

2. **Use concentrate/vape for symptoms of moderate to severe abdominal pain as needed.**

   While due to separate causes, patients with both IBS and IBD have acute episodes of pain, usually accompanied by GI symptoms. When severe pain hits, something that works quickly like vape is needed. Vape can be used at the onset of a bout of abdominal pain, especially when it is severe. Use a vape that is a concentrate from a cannabis strain that is particularly good for IBS or IBD (described above), which include White Widow, Harlequin, Durban Poison, and Cannatonic. When dosing a vape, start with one puff. Wait a few minutes until you feel an effect. You can increase the dose slowly, one puff at a time, until you feel relief from your abdominal pain, without feeling sleepy or high.

3. **If symptoms occur regularly (or to prevent regular symptoms), take pills/edibles or tincture several times a day with 2:1 or 1:1 ratio of CBD to THC.**

   With IBS, the cause is not known, but an endocannabinoid deficiency may be a factor that leads to neurotransmitter issues that causes pain and GI symptoms. For IBD, there is an autoimmune process that leads to inflammation that causes pain and GI symptoms. Thus, in both cases, there is a chronic condition that is always present. Thus, while CBD may help, and vape can help with acute pain, patients with IBS and IBD who have chronic daily symptoms should consider regular use of pills/edible or tinctures can help keep their pain and GI symptoms under control. Edibles last six to eight hours, and tinctures last four to six hours, so patients may need to take these remedies a few times a day. While edibles and tinctures come in a variety of ratios of CBD to THC (14:1, 4:1, 1:1, 1:4, et cetera), since I recommend that patients take higher doses of daily CBD, I have found it much easier (and less expensive) for patients to stick with 2:1 or 1:1 products. Since pills and tinctures are often reconstituted with terpenes added back, chose products specifically designed for pain, which have terpenes such as beta-caryophyllene and myrcene. While each state is different, some companies make edibles and tinctures that are either sativa, indica, or hybrid, and some companies even make strain-specific products, so you can use one of the strains listed above. Start with approximately 0.5 to 1 mg of THC for the first dose. You can figure out how much THC is in one pill or one dropperful of tincture by looking at the package. For example, a 2:1 tincture that comes in a 15-ml bottle with 300 mg cannabinoids, half a dropperful (0.5 ml or 10 drops) contains 10 mg of cannabinoids. So three drops will be about 2 mg of CBD and 1 mg THC. You can start with about 5 drops (1–2 mg of THC) each day, or even with each dose, and then slowly increase the amount of THC drop by drop until you get the desired amount of pain relief without side effects. Edibles are easier to dose because the milligrams are stated on the package, and you can usually easily cut an edible in half or quarter to achieve your desired dose. Most patients achieve good results at 2 to 10 mg of THC per dose.

Chapter 22 Notes

1. Lovell, R. M., and A. C. Ford. Global prevalence of and risk factors for irritable bowel syndrome: a metaanalysis. *Clin Gastroenterol Hepatol* 2012: 10, 712–721, e4.

2. Sultan, S., and A. Malhotra. Irritable Bowel Syndrome. *Ann Int Med* 2016: 166(11), ITC82–ITC95.

3. Ford, A., B. E. Lacy, L. A. Harris, et al. Effect of Antidepressants and Psychological Therapies in Irritable Bowel Syndrome: An Updated Systematic Review and Meta-Analysis. *Am J Gastro January* 2019: 114(1), 21–39.

4. Heenan, P. E., J. I. Keenan, S. Bayer, et al. Irritable bowel syndrome and the gut microbiota, *Journal of the Royal Society of New Zealand* 2019: DOI: 10.1080/03036758.2019.1695635.

5. Craig, O. New therapies in Irritable Bowel Syndrome: what works and when. *Curr Opin Gastroenterol* 2018: 34, 50–56.

6. Inflammatory Bowel Disease (Overview). https://my.clevelandclinic.org/health/diseases/15587-inflammatory-bowel-disease-overview. Accessed 5/16/20.

7. Russo, E. Clinical endocannabinoid deficiency (CECD): can this concept explain therapeutic benefits of cannabis in migraine, fibromyalgia, irritable bowel syndrome and other treatment-resistant conditions? *Neuro Endocrinol Lett* 2008 Apr: 29(2), 192–200.

8. Ahmed, W., and S. Katz. Therapeutic Use of Cannabis in Inflammatory Bowel Disease. *Gastroenterol Hepatol (NY)* 2016 Nov: 12(11), 668–679.

9. Lahat, A., A. Lang, and S. Ben-Horin. Impact of cannabis treatment on the quality of life, weight and clinical disease activity in inflammatory bowel disease patients: a pilot prospective study. *Digestion* 2012: 85(1), 1–8.

10. Bergamaschi, M. M., R. H. Queiroz, et al. Cannabidiol reduces the anxiety induced by simulated public speaking in treatment-naïve social phobia patients. *Neuropsychopharmacology* 2011 May: 36(6), 1219–26.

11. Shannon, S., et al. Cannabidiol in Anxiety and Sleep: A Large Case Series. *Perm J* 2019: 23, 18–041.

12. Xiong, W., T. Cui, et al. Cannabinoids suppress inflammatory and neuropathic pain by targeting α3 glycine receptors. *J Exp Med* 2012 Jun 4: 209(6), 1121–1134.

13. Philpott, H. T., M. O'Brien, and J. J. McDougall. Attenuation of early phase inflammation by cannabidiol prevents pain and nerve damage in rat osteoarthritis. *Pain* 2017: 158(12), 2442–2451.

Chapter 23:

How to Use Medical Cannabis and CBD for Nausea and Vomiting

Nausea and Vomiting

Nausea is the sensation that one might vomit, and vomiting itself is the expulsion of the contents of the stomach. Nausea and vomiting are natural responses that are meant to protect the body from ingesting substances that might be harmful. However, especially if associated with a chronic condition, they can be incredibly bothersome. There are many causes of nausea and vomiting. They be broken down into brain related causes (injury, tumor, migraine, seizure, motion sickness), gastrointestinal related (blockage, inflammation of the pancreas/pancreatitis, ulcer), infectious (viral, bacterial, food poisoning), medication side effects (opioids, chemotherapy), or toxins (alcohol, arsenic, pesticides), and from certain underlying medical conditions that disturb the body's chemical balance (thyroid issues, pregnancy).[1] Even conditions like pain, anxiety, and stress can cause nausea and vomiting. In many cases, the symptoms go away relatively quickly and do not require treatment (i.e., you drink too much, you throw up, and then you feel better). However, in recurrent conditions like migraines, or long-lasting conditions like pregnancy or chemotherapy, symptoms become bothersome enough to require treatment. In addition to rehydration, most treatments involve medications that reduce nausea and vomiting. While many can be quite effective, sometimes they are not, especially in severe cases.

Medical Cannabis and CBD for Nausea and Vomiting

There is strong evidence to support the use of medical cannabis for nausea and vomiting. A report from the National Academy of Sciences that reviewed all of the existing research on use of medical cannabis for a variety of medical conditions found that the use of medical cannabis for nausea, specifically regarding nausea that is a side effect of cancer patients undergoing chemotherapy, was one of three areas where there was compelling evidence that medical cannabis was effective.[2] While there are many prescription medications that can be effective for nausea and vomiting, such as Zofran (ondansetron), they do not always work for nausea induced by cancer.[3] We know that at least THC is effective for nausea, as Marinol (dronabinol) is a prescription medication that is a synthetic form of THC and approved for patients with chemotherapy-induced nausea, even though dronabinol may not be much better than other conventional prescription medications.[4] Interestingly, likely due to the entourage effect of whole-plant medicine, medical cannabis appears to be more effective than dronabinol for chemotherapy-induced nausea.[5] Of note, one of the common conditions that cause nausea is pregnancy. While the effects of medical cannabis (generally much lower doses than recreational marijuana) has not really been studied, studies of recreational marijuana indicate that THC can affect fetal brain development and has been associated with adverse outcomes such as low birth rate.[6] Thus, I do not recommend the use of medical cannabis for nausea related to pregnancy.

Strains for Nausea and Vomiting

The cannabis plant contains many different substances (called cannabinoids) that have medicinal properties. In addition to THC (the component that can make you "high") and CBD (which does not make you high), there are substances called terpenes that give cannabis its smell and flavor. The combination and proportion of cannabinoids and terpenes will help determine which strains are best to treat symptoms of nausea and vomiting. Limonene is a terpene that is also found in citrus fruits that appears to be particularly effective for gastrointestinal-related issues. Myrcene is another terpene that can also be found in hops, mango, and lemongrass, and has muscle-relaxation properties, which may reduce issues related to nausea and vomiting. While strains with these terpenes can be effective for nausea and vomiting, every patient is different, so it may take some trial and error to determine which strain is the right strain for you. A few strains that patients have successfully used for nausea and vomiting include the following:

Sour Diesel and Jack Herer. These are both sativa strains that have a medium (15–20%) amount of THC, with very little (<1%) CBD. They are known to be good as mood elevators, and both have the terpene caryophyllene which is anti-inflammatory and also helpful with nerve issues, some of which can affect nausea and vomiting. Sour Diesel may be particularly helpful for nausea and vomiting as it is high in limonene.

Durban Poison is another pure sativa strain that is used to treat conditions such as anxiety, depression, and stress. It also contains a medium (14–19%) amount of THC, with very little (<1%) CBD. Its predominant terpene is terpinolene followed by myrcene.

Blue Dream and **OG Kush** are both sativa-predominant hybrid strains that have a medium (16–20%) amount of THC, with very little (<1%) CBD. Both contain myrcene as their predominant terpene, and OG Kush has some limonene, which is good for gastrointestinal issues.

Northern Lights is a myrcene-heavy indica strain that is generally used for acute pain, but has also been used successfully for nausea and vomiting in some patients. It has a medium amount (14–19%) of THC, and very little (<1%) CBD.

CBD for Nausea and Vomiting

While THC, the psychoactive component of medical cannabis, is extremely effective for nausea and vomiting, CBD alone may also be useful in treating nausea and vomiting. There are two ways to think about CBD in the treatment of nausea and vomiting. First is the direct effect of CBD. While there are no clinical trials of CBD alone in patients with nausea and vomiting, at least in animal models, it appears that low doses of CBD can reduce both nausea and vomiting, likely through interactions with serotonin receptors in the brain (a similar pathway to Zofran/ondansetron).[7] A second way CBD can help with nausea and vomiting is by treating the underlying condition causing the nausea and vomiting. For example, seizures can lead to nausea and vomiting, and there is a substantial amount of research on CBD in the treatment of seizures, with Epidiolex being a cannabis-based, CBD-only product approved by the FDA for the treatment of seizures. One problem is that while CBD generally has no side effects, high doses of CBD cause nausea and vomiting. Thus, when using CBD as part of a medical cannabis regimen for nausea and vomiting, attention to dosage (which is usually not an issue for CBD) is warranted.

Using Different Formulations for Nausea and Vomiting

Almost as important as which strain of cannabis you use, or the ratio of THC to CBD, is the formulation you use to treat nausea and vomiting. This is because different formulations have different onsets of actions and different durations. Nausea and vomiting often come on suddenly and therefore require a formation that had a rapid onset of action (works in seconds or minutes). However, for chronic conditions that cause nausea and vomiting, or where symptoms may be prolonged, such as after chemotherapy, something that lasts a long time may be a better option.

Vape is probably the best and most common option for sudden onset of nausea and vomiting. Vape comes in the form of a concentrated liquid (called "**concentrate**") that is extracted from the cannabis plant, and usually heated so it can be inhaled. Vape also works very quickly (seconds to minutes), which is beneficial for nausea and vomiting. However, it also does not last very long (an hour or so), meaning that any sedation or other effects will disappear quickly, so you can get back to your day. Almost all cannabis strains come in vape or concentrate, so you can choose one of those listed above (or similar) to start with.

Tinctures are liquids that come in droppers. You drop tinctures under your tongue to allow for fast absorption rather than swallowing them directly. Tinctures take about thirty minutes to work and last four to six hours, so they can be excellent for chronic or longer-lasting conditions that cause nausea and vomiting. Tinctures are also slightly easier to titrate (adjust the dose), as they can be increased drop by drop. Finally, while this varies state by state, while most tinctures are extractions of primarily THC and CBD, some tinctures are available in sativa, indica, or hybrid strains, and some states sell extracts of the whole cannabis plant, so you can use a specific strain, like the ones listed above.

Pills or capsules (edibles) take a bit longer to work (one to two hours) but last longer in the body (up to eight hours), so they can be an excellent choice for chronic conditions that cause nausea and vomiting. Depending on the state, some edibles may be available as an indica, sativa, or hybrid and may even be available in a specific strain.

General Recommendations for Nausea and Vomiting

Since there are so many causes of nausea and vomiting, it is hard to make specific recommendations for every situation. However, in general patients are usually treating sudden onset of nausea and vomiting or are treating/preventing nausea or vomiting associated with chronic conditions or side effects from medications, like chemotherapy. The other aspect of nausea and vomiting is treating the underlying conditions that cause nausea and vomiting.

1. **Use concentrate/vape at the onset of nausea and vomiting.**
   Vape should be used at the onset of nausea and vomiting, especially when symptoms are severe. Also, if nausea and vomiting associated with medication, including chemotherapy does not last long, vape can be used prior to medication, as well as an hour or so later if needed. If symptoms last longer than a few hours, tinctures or edibles by themselves or in combination with vape may be preferred.

I recommend starting with a vape that is a concentrate from a cannabis strain that is particularly good for nausea and vomiting (as listed above), which include Sour Diesel, Jack Herer, Durban Poison, Blue Dream, OG Kush, and Northern Lights. When dosing a vape, start with one puff. Wait a few minutes until you feel an effect. You can increase the dose slowly, one puff at a time, until you feel relief from your nausea without feeling sleepy or high.

2. **Take pills/edibles or tinctures several times a day with a 2:1 or 1:1 ratio of CBD to THC for constant nausea or vomiting, either regularly or as needed.**

   Some patients have nausea and vomiting that last for hours, or they even experience them daily. Thus, the regular use of pills/edible or tinctures can help keep nausea and vomiting under control, or if taken daily, can even be preventative. Edibles last six to eight hours, and tinctures last four to six hours, so patients may need to take these remedies a few times a day. While edibles and tinctures come in a variety of ratios of CBD to THC (14:1, 4:1, 1:1, 1:4, et cetera), I have found it much easier (and less expensive) for patients to stick with 2:1 or 1:1 products, and then supplement with separate, hemp-based CBD if needed. Since pills and tinctures are often reconstituted with terpenes added back, choose products specifically designed for nausea, which have terpenes such as limonene and myrcene. While each state is different, some companies make edibles and tinctures that are either sativa, indica, or hybrid, and some companies even make strain-specific products, so you can use one of the strains listed above. Start with approximately 0.5 to 1 mg of THC for the first dose. You can figure out how much THC is in one pill or one dropperful of tincture by looking at the package. For example, a 2:1 tincture that comes in a 15-ml bottle with 300 mg cannabinoids, half a dropperful (0.5 ml or 10 drops) contains 10 mg of cannabinoids. So three drops will be about 2 mg of CBD and 1 mg THC. You can start with about five drops (1–2 mg of THC) each day, or even with each dose, and then slowly increase the amount of THC drop by drop until you get the desired amount of relief without side effects. Edibles are easier to dose because the milligrams are stated on the package, and you can usually easily cut an edible in half or quarter to achieve your desired dose. Most patients achieve good results at 2 to 10 mg of THC per dose.

3. **Use daily CBD capsule pill or tincture to treat underlying conditions and/or nausea itself, but start with lower doses.** CBD alone has a role in many underlying conditions that cause nausea (seizures, migraines, anxiety, IBS, et cetera). In addition, low doses of CBD alone can help treat nausea. However, while CBD has little side effects, high doses of CBD can rarely cause nausea and vomiting. Thus, I recommend starting with no more than 15 mg of CBD a day to ensure that CBD is helping and not making nausea and vomiting worse. This can either be a cannabis-derived CBD or pure-hemp-derived CBD. I generally recommend hemp-derived CBD, as it is less expensive and easier to obtain, and because there is virtually no THC, it will not make you sleepy or high.

Chapter 23 Notes

1. Scorza, K., A. Williams, J. D. Phillps, and J. Shaw. Evaluation of Nausea and Vomiting. *Am Fam Physician* 2007 Jul 1: 76(1), 76–84.

2. National Academies of Sciences, Engineering, and Medicine. 2017. The Health Effects of Cannabis and Cannabinoids: The Current State of Evidence and Recommendations for Research. Washington, DC: The National Academies Press. https://doi.org/10.17226/24625.

3. Ranganath, R., L. Einhorn, and C. Albany. Management of Chemotherapy Induced Nausea and Vomiting in Patients on Multiday Cisplatin Based Combination Chemotherapy. *Biomed Res Int* 2015: 943618.

4. Smith, L. A., F. Azariah, T. C. V. Lavender, N. S. Stoner, and S. Bettiol. 2015. Cannabinoids for nausea and vomiting in adults with cancer receiving chemotherapy. *Cochrane Databaseof Systematic Reviews* (11):CD009464.

5. Mortimer, T. L., T. Mabin, and A. Engelbrecht. Cannabinoids: the lows and the highs of chemotherapy-induced nausea and vomiting. *Future Oncology* 2019: 15(9), 1035–1049.

6. Crume et al: Cannabis use during the perinatal period in a state with legalized recreational and medical marijuana: the association between maternal characteristics, breastfeeding patterns, and neonatal outcomes. *J Pediatr* 2018: 197, 90–96.

7. Parker, L. A., E. M. Rock, and C. L. Limebeer. Regulation of nausea and vomiting by cannabinoids. *Br J Pharmacol* 2011 Aug: 163(7), 1411–1422.

Chapter 24:

How to Use Medical Cannabis and CBD in Cancer

Cancer may be the single most important disease where medical cannabis can help afflicted patients. Not only is there robust research for treating chemotherapy-induced nausea, but there is also promising early research for treating and even preventing cancer. More importantly, cancer is often fatal. Thus, concerns that some have about the potential harms and lack of research regarding using marijuana medicinally must be thrown out the window when a patient is dying. At its core, medical cannabis can relieve suffering, and cancer may be the one condition where relief of suffering is needed the most. There are essentially four ways to think about medical cannabis in patients with cancer: treating the symptoms of cancer, treating the side effects from cancer treatment, treating the cancer itself, and preventing cancer.

Treating Cancer Symptoms

There are many types of cancer, each with different associated symptoms. However, in general, cancer symptoms can be relieved by using medical cannabis. When cancer spreads locally, invading other organs, it can cause pain in the organ where the cancer has spread. When cancer metastasizes, it can travel to many places, very commonly the bones causing bone pain. Fortunately, medical cannabis is very good at treating pain, and has shown to be helpful in treating pain related to cancer.[1, 2, 3] Anxiety is also commonly associated with cancer. Patients are understandably anxious about the consequences of cancer. Also, in patients who are dying, anxiety is a common symptom. Medical cannabis is also good at alleviating anxiety (see Chapter 13) and has been shown to be helpful in patients with cancer-related anxiety.[4] Finally, patients with cancer often have issues with wasting and appetite. Growing cancer cells consume large amounts of energy, causing patients to lose weight, even with normal eating, and cancer cells produce chemical messengers that cause a decrease in appetite. Cannabis has been shown to improve appetite and decrease wasting.[5,6]

Treating the Side Effects of Cancer Treatments

There are many forms of cancer treatment, including surgery and radiation, but chemotherapy tends to be associated with the most significant amount of side effects. Chemotherapy essentially works by poisoning cells, with the hopes that the treatment can kill the cancer cells without hurting too many normal cells along the way. Not surprisingly, many patients do not feel well when getting chemotherapy. Nausea is a common side effect from chemotherapy. Fortunately, the data on medical cannabis successfully treating chemotherapy-induced nausea is robust, and the review by the National Academies of Sciences concluded that medical cannabis was effective for this.[7] Another common and disabling side effect from chemotherapy is neuropathy. Neuropathy is the sensation of tingling and pain caused by damage to nerve cells. It occurs most commonly in the extremities. While nausea usually resolves soon after a chemotherapy cycle is complete, postchemotherapy neuropathy can persist and sometimes may even become permanent. Because of the concentration of CB1 receptors on nerve cells, medical cannabis can be effective in treating and possibly even preventing postchemotherapy neuropathy.

Treating the Cancer Itself

In addition to treating cancer symptoms and side effects from treatment, medical cannabis may be useful for actually treating the cancer itself. Research has shown that cannabinoids like THC and CBD affect cancer cells very differently than normal, healthy cells. Cannabis has been shown in laboratory studies to turn on switches that cause cancer cells to die, prevent cancer cells from metastasizing, limit the growth of cancer cells, and prevent a process called angiogenesis, which is where cancer cells make their own blood vessels to help them get nourishment and grow.[8, 9, 10] While there are sporadic reports of patients using cannabis alone to treat their cancer successfully,[11, 12] there is not sufficient data to recommend this medically as an approach to treat cancer with cannabis alone. However, using cannabis along with chemotherapy can be done safely, and research has shown that using cannabis with typical cancer treatments can be more effective and causes fewer side effects than just using typical cancer treatments alone.[13] One form of cancer treatment is immunotherapy, which uses elements of the body's immune system to fight cancer. Since cannabis can be anti-inflammatory, using medical cannabis during these types of treatment should be done with caution. Finally, there are some potential interactions with certain chemotherapeutic agents where doses may need adjusting, so using medical cannabis in consultation with an oncologist is strongly advised.

Prevention of Cancer

For the same reasons that cannabis is effective in treating cancer, it may be effective in preventing cancer. This area of research is still in the early stages, but there is some animal evidence suggesting that this may be possible. Mice can be bred to be predisposed to developing certain kinds of cancer. In two studies, one for colon cancer[14] and another for lung cancer,[15] mice who were predisposed to these cancers were much less likely to develop those cancers than mice that did not receive cannabis. It is unclear whether or not people unaffected by cancer should start using medical cannabis before they develop cancer. However, for patients at very high risk, including those patients who have been successfully treated for cancer and are concerned about recurrence, they might be excellent candidates. In addition, though research is extremely limited, CBD alone may have anticancer properties,[16] and because it is not psychoactive, it could be a reasonable option for anyone wanting to prevent cancer.

Strains for Cancer

It is well established that the different terpene profiles of various cannabis strains are an important component of how that particular cannabis strain affects the body. In fact, the terpene profile may be more important on these effects than the amount and ratio of THC and CBD in a given strain. However, while some strains may be better for nausea, and some strains may be better for neuropathy, there is simply not enough research to know which strains are better for cancer in general, let alone specific strains for specific types of cancer (e.g., best strains for prostate cancer versus best strains for breast cancer). In addition, because of the holistic nature of the whole plant, one strain of cannabis may help treating cancer symptoms, cancer-treatment-related effects, and the cancer itself. Thus, my general recommendations for specific strains are related to both the symptoms related to cancer and the effects of cancer treatment, and are not cancer-type specific. Some examples include the following:

Blue Dream is a sativa-predominant hybrid strain that has a medium (16–20%) amount of THC, with very little (<1%) CBD. It has myrcene as its predominant terpene, which can help with relaxation, and can be particularly good with nausea.

Harlequin is another a sativa-dominant hybrid but has a much higher CBD-to-THC ratio (5:2, with about 4–7% THC, 8–16% CBD); it is also high in myrcene. Harlequin is an excellent option for pain relief during the day, as it tends not to be as sedating.

White Widow is a hybrid strain that has about 20% THC and 1% CBD that works well for all types of pain (bone pain, neuropathic pain). It is also good for anxiety associated with cancer.

ACDC is also a hybrid strain, which, like White Widow, is good for both pain and anxiety. However, it's known for having low levels of THC. It has the opposite ratio of White Widow, with a 20:1 CBD-to-THC ratio. Thus, this is one strain that should not make you "high."

Granddaddy Purple (GDP) is a pure indica that has a medium (15–19%) amount of THC, with very little (<1%) CBD. GDP has myrcene and caryophyllene as its terpenes and can be useful in both anxiety and insomnia, which can be seen in patients with cancer.

Northern Lights is another pure indica, like GDP, with a medium (14–19%) amount of THC, and very little (<1%) CBD. Its predominant terpenes are myrcene and caryophyllene. Like GDP, it is also useful for insomnia and anxiety, which is seen in cancer. In addition, Northern Lights can be useful in nausea.

CBD for Cancer

CBD is the nonpsychoactive cannabinoid in medical cannabis and is also found in hemp. CBD is known to be effective for anxiety (see Chapter 6 and Chapter 13), which, as previously mentioned, is commonly seen in patients with cancer. CBD also has anti-inflammatory properties, which may play a role in the treatment of cancer itself. While there is plenty of research (mostly in animal studies but a few human clinical trials as well) that suggests the cannabinoids, particularly THC, can play a role in cancer treatment, the role of CBD alone (either cannabis derived or hemp derived) in treating cancer is very limited. There are several research studies showing that CBD can increase the rate at which cancer cells die, as well as prevent cancer cells from spreading,[17] and even some preliminary data in human patients with cancer showing benefit.[16] While there may be limited evidence of using CBD to treat cancer, in addition to helping with anxiety, CBD also mitigates some of the unwanted effects of THC, particularly feeling "high" or sleepy. Thus, there are several good reasons to consider CBD to be part of an overall regimen in patients with cancer.

However, there are two areas to consider where using CBD in patients with should be done with caution. The first is interaction with chemotherapeutic agents. While drug-drug interactions are relatively minimal for both THC and CBD, CBD at high doses can either increase or decrease the effectiveness of medications, including chemotherapy. This is important because if the dose of chemotherapy is too high, it may cause unwanted side effects, and if the dose is too low, it may not be as effective. Thus, if using CBD in combination with chemotherapy, especially high-dose CBD, consultation with an oncologist is strongly recommended. The second area is anorexia and wasting. Patients with cancer can have decreased appetite and weight loss. THC is quite good at helping with this, but CBD, particularly at high doses, could have the opposite effect.

While CBD-only products can be derived from either marijuana or hemp, I generally recommend hemp-derived CBD because it is usually less expensive, and you can obtain this without certification. However, because hemp-derived CBD is not regulated by the FDA, you must be very careful that you are getting a high-quality, full-spectrum, third-party-verified product. If you decide to try CBD in patients with cancer, I recommend no more than 25 mg to 30 mg of CBD a day, which can be obtained by using CBD oil/tincture under the tongue, or CBD oil capsules. CBD, in general, does not immediately alleviate anxiety, or other symptoms related to cancer for that matter, but rather taken daily for at least one to two weeks, it can start to affect some of the chemical signaling in the brain to help alleviate anxiety and possibly help with other aspects of cancer symptoms or treatment-associated side effects.

Using Different Formulations for Cancer

Almost as important as which strain of cannabis you use, or the ratio of THC to CBD, is the formulation used to treat your cancer symptoms or treatment-related side effects. Some of this is due to the fact that different formulations have different onsets of actions and different durations. Some symptoms like pain may be constantly present and thus require a longer-acting agent, while some symptoms like nausea after chemotherapy may come on quickly and require a more rapid-acting agent.

Pills or capsules (edibles) take longer to work (about an hour), but last longer in the body (up to eight hours), so edibles are excellent options for symptoms that are present all day, which can include pain or anxiety. In addition, edibles are quite easy to use and therefore may be preferred by cancer patients who are very ill. Depending on the state, some edibles may be available as an indica, sativa, or hybrid and may even be available in a specific strain.

Tinctures are liquids that come in droppers. You place drops of tincture under your tongue to allow for fast absorption, rather than swallowing them directly. Tinctures take about thirty minutes to work and last four to six hours. There are two advantages for using tinctures in patients with cancer. The first is that they are generally easier to titrate (slowly adjust) the dose, since doses can be increased drop by drop. This is particularly important for very ill patients, as doses should be started at very low and slowly increased to prevent side effects. Secondly, for patients with cancer who are severely ill or debilitated, tinctures may also be easier for caregivers to give patients who may not be able to swallow edibles and/or use vapes. Finally, while this varies state by state, while most tinctures are extractions of primarily THC and CBD, some tinctures are available in sativa, indica, or hybrid strains, and some states sell extracts of the whole cannabis plant, so you can use a specific strain, like the ones listed above.

Vape commonly comes in the form of a concentrated liquid (called "**concentrate**") that is extracted from the cannabis plant, and usually heated so it can be inhaled. Vape also works very quickly (in seconds to minutes), which is very beneficial for acute and severe symptoms. This can be particularly good for something like severe nausea, or patients who need something to help them fall asleep. However, it also doesn't last very long (an hour or so), meaning that vape alone is probably not practical for something that is present all the time, such as chronic pain. Almost all cannabis strains come in vape or concentrate, so you can choose one of those listed above (or similar) to start with.

Topical agents can be applied primarily for localized areas related to pain. One advantage of topical agents is that there is little absorption into the bloodstream, so even if a cream or salve you are using has a high amount of THC, it won't make you sleepy or high. Topical agents can be expensive to use, so I only recommend them where there is a specific part in the body that is painful and thus does not requiring a large amount of cream. Topical agents usually last a few hours, so they require multiple applications a day.

General Recommendations for Using Medical Cannabis and CBD in Patients with Cancer

Since medical cannabis and CBD can treat symptoms related to the disease and its treatment, as well as treat the disease itself, cannabinoids have a potentially important role in patients with cancer. Another benefit of plant-based medicine is that since cannabis has multiple agents (as opposed to a single molecule used in a typical prescription), several symptoms can be treated simultaneously. Thus, there is no one single way to use cannabis in patients with cancer. Rather, each treatment regimen should be customized to a patient's particular symptoms or cancer-related issues. Patients should use medical cannabis with caution if using immunotherapy as a treatment, and in general, I always recommend consulting with an oncologist, especially since cannabis may interact with certain cancer chemotherapies.

1. **Take daily medium- to high-dose CBD.** Since cannabis can be effective for both cancer treatment and prevention, in my opinion, it makes sense that any patient diagnosed with cancer (or even at high risk) should be using cannabinoids on a regular basis. Thus, in addition to taking medical cannabis to treat cancer symptoms and treatment side effects, I recommend that patients supplement their regimen with 15 mg to up to 30 mg of hemp-derived CBD daily using the lower end for use in patients with wasting/weight loss or whose cancer chemotherapy could have an interaction with CBD. When cancer symptoms

or treatment side effects have abated, patients can continue to take 25 to 30 mg of CBD regularly, as there may be a role in preventing a recurrence.

2. **Treat cancer symptoms, focusing on the most predominant symptom first**. Patient with cancer will likely have multiple symptoms at once, in addition to treatment-related side effects (see below). Fortunately, cannabis can treat several things at once. Thus, it is usually best to first focus on the most severe symptom, as other minor symptoms might improve as a result. When considering treatment, try to choose appropriate strains as well as formulations that match the need for either rapid onset of action or something that lasts throughout the day or night.

   a. **Pain:** If pain is chronic, or occurring all the time, edibles with higher ratios of THC should be used (e.g., 1:1 tablets two to three times a day). Start with a small dose (e.g., half a 5 mg tablet), and slowly increase with each day until pain has diminished without sedation. For more acute or severe pain, a more rapid-acting concentrate or vape may be needed. ACDC is a good hybrid strain for pain. Harlequin is another sativa-dominant strain that can be used for pain during the day with less sedation. Both vape and edibles can be used together if pain is chronic with severe or acute exacerbations.

   b. **Anxiety:** Using CBD as recommended above should help to some degree with anxiety, though this will usually take one to two weeks to have a significantly noticeable effect. If anxiety is constant throughout the day, using an edible (as suggested for pain) may be quite effective. However, for acute bouts of anxiety, a more rapid-acting concentrate or vape can be helpful—either a hybrid strain like White Widow, or an indica strain such as Granddaddy Purple or Northern Lights. In addition, patients with anxiety tend to have issues with sleep. A pill or tincture with a high level of THC and another cannabinoid called CBN prior to bedtime can help. There are several companies that produce tinctures and edibles with a 1:1 THC-to-CBN ratio and some also contain natural ingredients such as chamomile and melatonin that can be quite effective to help induce sleep.

c. **Wasting:** THC is the component of cannabis that gives recreational users the "munchies," which is why medical cannabis can be helpful for wasting and loss of appetite. Indica strains like Granddaddy Purple are high in THC and can be helpful in stimulating appetite. Patients can use either tinctures or vape/concentrate, before meals.

3. **Treat cancer-treatment-related side effects:** There are two ways to combat chemotherapy side effects with medical cannabis: pretreatment to prevent the side effects, and actual treatment of the side effects.

a. **Nausea induced by chemotherapy:** THC is a potent reliever of nausea. Using a high-THC or THC-only product is best to prevent and treat nausea. For pretreatment, patients can use edibles at least forty-five to sixty minutes prior to treatment. For nausea symptoms, immediate relief is usually necessary, and using a vape/concentrate is usually necessary. Ideally, use a strain that is particularly good for nausea at the onset of symptoms. Start with one puff, and gradually increase the dose until nausea is relieved without feeling sedation or "high." Two good strains for nausea include Northern Lights (a high-indica strain), or Blue Dream (a sativa strain).

b. **Peripheral neuropathy:** Both THC and CBD can be good for peripheral neuropathy. Taking daily CBD as recommended should already help for this. For additional benefit, low doses of edibles (e.g., 1:1 CBD: THC) can be taken at least forty-five to sixty minutes prior to treatment. For treatment of symptoms, patients experience peripheral neuropathy differently. Some patients perceive this as a chronic, dull burning, usually in the extremities, while other perceive this as sharp and severe pain. For more chronic pain, using edibles or tinctures a few times a day can be helpful. For acute, severe pain, use concentrate/vape as needed, using strains particularly good for neuropathic pain, such as White Widow or ACDC.

Chapter 24 Notes

1. Johnson, J. R., M. Burnell-Nugent, D. Lossignol, et al. Multicenter, double-blind, randomized, placebo-controlled, parallel-group study of the efficacy, safety, and tolerability of THC:CBD extract and THC extract in patients with intractable cancer-related pain. *J Pain Symptom Manage* 2010 Feb: 39(2), 167–79.

2. Portenoy, R. K., et al. Nabiximols for opioid-treated cancer patients with poorly-controlled chronic pain: a randomized, placebo-controlled, graded-dose trial. *The Journal of Pain* 2012: 13(5), 438–449.

3. Teoh, D., T. J. Smith, M. Song, and N. M. Spirtos. Care After Chemotherapy: Peripheral Neuropathy, Cannabis for Symptom Control, and Mindfulness. *Am Soc Clin Oncol Educ Book* 2018 May 23: 38, 469–479.

4. Regelson, W., J. R. Butler, J. Schulz, T. Kirk, L. Peek, M. L. Green, and M. O. Zalis. Delta 9-THC as an effective antidepressant and appetite-stimulating agent in advanced cancer patients. In M. C. Braude and S. Szara (Eds.), *The Pharmacology of Marihuana* (pp. 763–776). New York: Raven Press, 1976.

5. Abrams, D. I., and M. Guzman. Cannabis in cancer care. *Clinical Pharmacology & Therapeutics* 2015: 97(6), 575–586.

6. Jatoi, A., H. E. Windschitl, C. L. Loprinzi, et al. Dronabinol versus megestrol acetate versus combination therapy for cancer-associated anorexia: a North Central Cancer Treatment Group study. *J Clin Oncol* 2002 Jan 15: 20(2), 567–73.

7. National Academies of Sciences, Engineering, and Medicine. 2017. The Health Effects of Cannabis and Cannabinoids: The Current State of Evidence and Recommendations for Research. Washington, DC: The National Academies Press.

8. Munson, A. E., L. S. Harris, M. A. Friedman, W. L. Dewey, and R. A. Carchman. Antineoplastic Activity of Cannabinoids. *JNCI: Journal of the National Cancer Institute* 1975 September: 55(3), 597–602.

9. National Toxicology Program. NTP Toxicology and Carcinogenesis

Studies of 1-Trans-Delta(9)-Tetrahydrocannabinol (CAS No. 1972-08-3) in F344 Rats and B6C3F1 Mice (Gavage Studies). *Natl Toxicol Program Tech Rep Ser* 1996 Nov: 446, 1–317.

10. Ladin, D. A., et al. Preclinical and clinical assessment of cannabinoids as anti-cancer agents. *Frontiers in pharmacology* 2016: 7, 361.

11. Singh, Y., and C. Bali. Cannabis Extract Treatment for Terminal Acute Lymphoblastic Leukemia with a Philadelphia Chromosome Mutation. *Case reports in oncology* 2013: 6(3), 585–592.

12. Kander, J. *Cannabis for the Treatment of Cancer: The Anticancer Activity of Phytocannabinoids and Endocannabinoids*, 4th edition, 2017.

13. Galve-Roperh, I., C. Sánchez, M. L. Cortés, T. Gómez del Pulgar, M. Izquierdo, and M. Guzmán. Anti-tumoral action of cannabinoids: involvement of sustained ceramide accumulation and extracellular signal-regulated kinase activation. *Nat Med* 2000 Mar: 6(3), 313–9.

14. Aviello, G., B. Romano, F. Borrelli, et al. Chemopreventive effect of the non-psychotropic phytocannabinoid cannabidiol on experimental colon cancer. *J Mol Med (Berl)* 2012 Aug: 90(8), 925–34.

15. Preet, A., R. K. Ganju, Groopman, J. E. Delta9-Tetrahydrocannabinol inhibits epithelial growth factor-induced lung cancer cell migration in vitro as well as its growth and metastasis in vivo. *Oncogene* 2008 Jan 10: 27(3), 339–46.

16. Kenyon, J., W. Liu, and A. Dalgleish. Report of objective clinical responses of cancer patients to pharmaceutical-grade synthetic cannabidiol. *Anticancer research* 2018: 38(10), 5831–5835.

17. Massi, P., et al. Cannabidiol as potential anticancer drug. *British journal of clinical pharmacology* 2013: 75(2), 303–312.

Chapter 25:

How to Use Medical Cannabis and CBD to Treat Male Sexual Disorders (ED)

Male Sexual Disorders

Until 1998, when Viagra came to market with US senator and war hero Bob Dole as its pitchman, erectile dysfunction (ED) was rarely discussed in the examination room, while many men suffered in silence. First, treatment options prior to medications like sildenafil (Viagra) did not work that well and were difficult to use. Second, men were not comfortable discussing this subject, even with their doctor. Shortly thereafter Viagra become one of the fastest-growing prescription medications in history, and men were eager to ask their physicians for prescriptions. I can personally attest to multiple conversations with patients, usually at the end of a visit, that started with, "By the way, doc…" and quickly turned for a request for that "little blue pill." While sildenafil and similar medications have helped many men, they do not work for everyone, there are some side effects, and there are restrictions for patients on certain heart medications. Another common sexual disorder in men is premature ejaculation (PE). This can be similarly embarrassing for men to discuss, and unlike ED, pharmaceutical treatment options are extremely limited.

Medical Cannabis for Male Sexual Disorders

Fortunately, medical cannabis may be helpful for both ED and PE. Research is, not surprisingly, extremely limited. In addition, there is some controversy regarding whether medical cannabis can be helpful or even possibly lead to male sexual disorders. On the one hand, survey studies done in both men and women suggest that sex is better when using marijuana prior to sexual activities, with reasons including increased desire, increased sensitivity, and increased relaxation.[1] On the other hand, reviews of multiple studies suggest that ED may be twice as common in those who use cannabis than those that do not.[2] Looking at mechanism of action, an erection is caused by an increase in blood flow to the penis. At least in animal studies, there is some evidence that THC[3] can dilate blood vessels, though this has not been researched specifically in humans or in the blood vessels involved in an erection.

While studies are again limited, there are likely many reasons for this conflicting evidence. First, there is clear evidence that cigarette smoking is linked to ED.[4] While nicotine may be one factor, there are other factors related to smoking itself. Thus, formulation (smoking versus vaping) may play a large role. Second, many of these studies associating ED with cannabis use investigated regular recreational marijuana use, which is different than using medical cannabis to treat a disease. Recreationally used marijuana also tends to use higher amounts of THC. We know that high doses of THC can cause anxiety, while lower doses can relieve anxiety, so this may play a role in ED and PE as well. Finally, both ED and PE have many causes; stress and anxiety are important ones. Thus, the ability of medical cannabis to increase relaxation may be the main reason why it is effective in both conditions, which seem to be opposite in nature. Other causes of sexual disfunction, particularly ED, in males include nerve damage and decreased blood flow. Thus, different strains might be used for different causes.

Strains for Male Sexual Disorders

Cannabis contains many different substances (called cannabinoids) that have medicinal properties. In addition to THC (the component that can make you "high") and CBD (which does not make you high), there are substances called terpenes that give cannabis its smell and flavor. The combination and proportion of cannabinoids and terpenes will help determine which strains are best to treat sexual problems. While there are no randomized studies that have compared the various strains of cannabis plants and have determined which is the most effective for sexual problems, indica-based strains, which tend to be more relaxing and sedating, tend to work best.

One terpene that seems to play an important role in sexual dysfunction is myrcene. Myrcene can also be found in hops, mango, and lemongrass. It has muscle-relaxation properties and can also help with pain, which could be a factor in sexual functioning. While there are several strains that have been reported to help with male sexual disorders, every patient is different, so it may take some trial and error to determine which strain is the right strain for you. A few strains that patients have successfully used for male sexual disorders include the following:

Green Crack is a sativa strain that has a medium (15–19%) amount of THC, with very little (<1%) CBD. It contains the terpene caryophyllene, which is useful in neve pain as well as depression.

Blue Dream is a sativa-predominant hybrid strain that has a medium (16–20%) amount of THC, with very little (<1%) CBD. It has myrcene as its predominant terpene, which can help with relaxation.

Blue Knight is a balanced hybrid, being about 50% sativa and 50% indica. It also has high amounts (27%) of THC, with low, but relevant, amounts (4%) of CBD.

Golden Strawberry is an indica-dominant hybrid known for its arousing and relaxing effects and known to treat erectile dysfunction. This is a high (20–23%) amount of THC, with very little (<1%) CBD. There is also close to 1% CBG. Golden Strawberry is high in limonene, making it uplifting. It also has a fair amount of myrcene, which is helpful for relaxation.

Granddaddy Purple (GDP) is a pure indica that has a medium (15–19%) amount of THC, with very little (<1%) CBD. GDP has myrcene and caryophyllene as its terpenes and can be useful in ED and PE for its relaxing and sedating properties.

CBD for Male Sexual Disorders

CBD is the nonpsychoactive cannabinoid in medical cannabis and is also found in hemp. While combinations of both THC and CBD can be effective for a variety of conditions, including sexual dysfunction, there is much less evidence that CBD alone can be helpful to treat male sexual disorders. However, there are several reasons that CBD by itself may be effective for both ED and PE. Both of these conditions can be associated with anxiety, and there is evidence that CBD is effective for general anxiety. While there are a few small studies that show that high-dose CBD might reduce acute anxiety before a stressful event, such as public speaking,[5] CBD has better evidence if taken on a daily basis, at lower doses (around 25 mg daily), to reduce general anxiety.[6]

There some other reasons why CBD may be effective in sexual disorders for men. Like THC, there is some extremely limited data that (at least in rats) CBD may dilate blood vessels, which is important to achieving and maintaining an erection.[7] In addition, likely due to damage they cause blood vessels throughout the body, both heart disease and diabetes are risk factors for ED. There is mounting evidence that CBD can be helpful for blood vessels and the cardiovascular system,[8] and it may even lower the risk of developing diabetes.[9]

While you can either use cannabis-derived CBD or hemp-derived CBD for daily treatment of anxiety, I generally recommend hemp-derived CBD because it is usually less expensive, and you can obtain this without certification. However, because hemp-derived CBD is not regulated by the FDA, you must be very careful that you are getting a high-quality, full-spectrum, third-party-verified product. For the treatment of male sexual disorders, I recommend 25 to 30 mg of CBD a day, which can be obtained by using CBD oil/tincture under the tongue, or CBD oil capsules. CBD, in general, does not immediately treat sexual dysfunction, but rather, taken daily for at least one to two weeks, it can start to affect some of the chemical signaling in the brain that may help to alleviate problems. Thus, don't expect to see improvement in symptoms right away.

Using Different Formulations for Sexual Dysfunction

Almost as important as which strain of cannabis you use, or the ratio of THC to CBD, is the formulation you use for sexual dysfunction. This is because different formulations have different onset of actions and different durations. Most sexual issues occur "in the moment." Thus, a rapid oneself of action (works in second or minutes) is likely going to be more effective. However, as mentioned, some sexual issues are due to conditions like stress or anxiety, which could be constantly present, and therefore best treated with something that lasts a long time.

Tinctures are liquids that come in droppers. You place drops of tincture under your tongue to allow for fast absorption, rather than swallowing them directly. Tinctures take about thirty minutes to work and last four to six hours. Tinctures are also generally easier to titrate (slowly adjust) the dose, since doses can be increased drop by drop. Tinctures are often available in a variety of ratios of CBD to THC, which allows for further customization of balancing improvement in sexual function with sedation or getting "high." In addition, while this varies state by state, though most tinctures are extractions of primarily THC and CBD, some tinctures are available in sativa, indica, or hybrid strains, and some states sell extracts of the whole cannabis plant, so you can use a specific strain like the ones listed above.

Pills or capsules (edibles) take a bit longer to work (one to two hours), but last longer in the body (up to eight hours), so they can be an excellent choice for something that may be contributing to ED or PE, like anxiety. However, unlike Viagra, this is not a pill you want to take prior to sexual activity, as it may take too long to start working. Depending on the state, some edibles may be available as an indica, sativa, or hybrid and may even be available in a specific strain.

Vape comes in the form of a concentrated liquid (called "**concentrate**") that is extracted from the marijuana plant, and usually heated so it can be inhaled. Vape also works very quickly (seconds to minutes), which is very beneficial for sexual disorders, as they often occur in the moment. However, it also doesn't last very long (an hour or so), meaning that any sedation or other effects will disappear quickly. Almost all cannabis strains come in vape or concentrate, so you can choose one of those listed above (or similar) to start with.

Topical formulations of medical cannabis come in salves and balms. One general advantage of topicals is that despite some having high amounts of THC, because they are applied to the skin, very little is absorbed in the bloodstream, and thus topical formulations have no psychoactive properties. However, balms or creams take more than a few minutes to work, so they may not be the best option for sexual disorders. In addition, the male genitals are highly vascular, and even though topicals generally have a low rate of absorption, this could potentially lead to side effects and is why almost every prescription or over-the-counter cream directs patients not to apply to genitals. Thus, I generally do not recommend topicals for male sexual disorders.

General Recommendations for Using Medical Cannabis and CBD in Men with Sexual Disorders

Because male sexual disorders can be very different (ED is very different from PE), and their causes are also diverse (stress, nerve damage, vascular problems), the best way to think about using medical cannabis and CBD for male sexual disorders is to first consider the underlying cause, and the select the appropriate cannabis treatment based on how the strain and/or formulation works to help with these issues. Finally, different people react differently to different strains and formulations of cannabis. In general, I recommend a "start low, go slow" approach, and the same is true for sexual disorders. Thus, it might take some time to find the right strain and right formulation to treat your sexual dysfunction; thus patience is warranted.

1. **For both ED and PE, use a vape fifteen to twenty minutes before anticipated sexual activity.**

   Vape is probably the best formulation for sexual dysfunction in men. It can be taken before sexual activity to help with both ED and PE. While everyone reacts differently to different strains, I would start with a hybrid strain like **Blue Knight** or an indica-leaning hybrid like **Golden Strawberry**. If vape is not preferred, tincture is also a good option, though (like Viagra and Cialis) you need to take it at least thirty minutes before sexual activity.

2. **Use daily CBD edibles (or tincture) if you have anxiety, and possibly diabetes or heart disease.**

   Again, it is unclear whether or not CBD alone can help with sexual issues in men. However, since we know it helps in anxiety, men who believe anxiety is a component of their sexual dysfunction should consider daily CBD. CBD may also decrease inflammation, increase blood flow, and reduce blood sugar—all of which can be contributing factors to ED. Thus, men with ED and heart disease and/or diabetes should consider daily CBD as well. I recommend 25 mg to 30 mg of CBD a day in a pill/edible/capsule or tincture. This can either be a marijuana-derived CBD or pure-hemp-derived CBD, though I generally recommend hemp-derived CBD, as it is less expensive and easier to obtain, and because there is virtually no THC, it will not make you sleepy or high.

3. **Consider nonpharmacological approaches to sexual dysfunction.**

   Sexual disorders are complex. Prior to Viagra, when there were limited treatments, many nonpharmacologic options were used and are still used today. In addition to vacuum devices and surgery for ED, there are various forms of counseling and behavior approaches than can help. While beyond the scope of this book, there are many therapists and other professionals who are experts in this area.

Chapter 25 Notes

1. Wiebe, E., and A. Just. How Cannabis Alters Sexual Experience: A Survey of Men and Women. *J Sex Med* 2019: 16, 1758–1762.

2. Pizzol, D., J. Demurtas, B. Stubbs, et al. Relationship Between Cannabis Use and Erectile Dysfunction: A Systematic Review and Meta-Analysis. *Am J Mens Health* 2019 Nov–Dec: 13(6).

3. Ellis, E. F., S. F. Moore, and K. A. Willoughby. Anandamide and delta 9-THC dilation of cerebral arterioles is blocked by indomethacin. *Am J Physiol Heart Circ Physiol* 1995: 269, H1859–64.

4. Kovac, J. R., C. Labbate, R. Ramasamy, et al. Effects of cigarette smoking on erectile dysfunction. *Andrologia* 2015 Dec: 47(10), 1087–1092.

5. Bergamaschi, M. M., R. H. Queiroz, et al. Cannabidiol reduces the anxiety induced by simulated public speaking in treatment-naïve social phobia patients. *Neuropsychopharmacology* 2011 May: 36(6), 1219–26.

6. Shannon, S., et al. Cannabidiol in Anxiety and Sleep: A Large Case Series. *Perm J* 2019: 23, 18–041.

7. Offertaler, L., F. M. Mo, S. Bátkai, et al. Selective ligands and cellular effectors of a G protein-coupled endothelial cannabinoid receptor. *Mol Pharmacol* 2003: 63, 699–705.

8. Stanley, C. P., W. H. Hind, and S. E. O'Sullivan. Is the cardiovascular system a therapeutic target for cannabidiol? *Br J Clin Pharmacol* 2012: 75(2), 313–322.

9. Weiss, L., M. Zeira, S. Reich, et al. Cannabidiol lowers incidence of diabetes in non-obese diabetic mice. *Autoimmunity* 2006 Mar: 39(2), 143–51.

Chapter 26:

How to Use Medical Cannabis and CBD to Treat Female Sexual Disorders

Female Sexual Disorders

When it comes to sexual disorders, in general, men are pretty simple, and women's issues can be rather complex. While low libido can be an issue for some men, especially those who are older or who have low testosterone, male sexual disorders primarily fall into two issues: erectile dysfunction (ED) or premature ejaculation (PE). In contrast, women can have many issues related to sexual function. Women can not only have low libido, but due to hormonal fluctuations, libido can go up and down. Women who are premenopausal can have issues related to menses, such as cramps, that can interfere with sexual activity, and low estrogen seen in women who are postmenopausal leads to a long list of ailments, including hot flashes and vaginal dryness, the latter of which can cause pain during sex (called dyspareunia). In addition, more often than men, these issues are connected (e.g., having pain during sex can lead to decreased desire to have sex). Finally, as of this writing, the "female Viagra" has yet to be discovered, so there are extremely limited pharmaceutical options for women with sexual disorders.

Medical Cannabis for Female Sexual Disorders

Fortunately, medical cannabis may be helpful for a variety of sexual disorders in women. Though research is extremely limited, there are some studies that look at medical cannabis and sexual function. Survey studies done in both men and women suggest that sex is better when using marijuana prior to sexual activities, with reasons including increased desire, increased sensitivity, and increased relaxation.[1] Another survey found that marijuana use seems to be correlated with an increase in sexual desire, as measured by frequency of having sex.[2] There are a few physiological reasons why this might be the case. First, oxytocin is an important hormone that reduces pain during labor and is increased during breastfeeding to stimulate milk production. It also is increased during orgasm. Research suggests that cannabis may be able to enhance the effects of oxytocin on the brain and thus improve orgasm.[3] Another mechanism of action could be increased blood flow. In men, the mechanism that causes an erection is through an increase in blood flow to the penis. While women do not have erections, increased blood flow to the vagina and surrounding tissues is important for arousal, lubrication, and sensitivity. At least in animal studies, there is some evidence that THC[4] can dilate blood vessels, though this has not been researched specifically in humans or in the blood vessels involved in erections or female arousal. While research on the benefits of medical cannabis in sexual dysfunction is very limited, there is at least one survey of 373 women, that of the 127 women who reported using marijuana before sex, the majority of these women reported increases in sex drive, improvement in orgasm, and a decrease in pain.[5] Finally, while there are many causes of sexual dysfunction in women, stress and anxiety often play an important role. We know that while high doses of THC can cause anxiety, lower doses can relieve anxiety, so relieving anxiety may play an important role in helping women with sexual function.

Strains for Female Sexual Disorders

Cannabis contains many different substances (called cannabinoids) that have medicinal properties. In addition to THC (the component that can make you "high") and CBD (which does not make you high), there are substances called terpenes that give cannabis its smell and flavor. The combination and proportion of cannabinoids and terpenes will help determine which strains are best to treat sexual problems. While there are no randomized studies that have compared the various strains of cannabis plants and have determined which is the most effective for female sexual problems, indica-based strains, which tend to be more relaxing and sedating, tend to work best.

One terpene that seems to play an important role in sexual dysfunction is myrcene. Myrcene can also be found in hops, mango, and lemongrass and has muscle-relaxation properties and can also help with pain, which could be a factor in sexual functioning. While there are several strains that have been reported to help with female sexual disorders, every patient is different, so it may take some trial and error to determine which strain is the right strain for you. A few strains that patients have successfully used for female sexual disorders include the following:

Green Crack is a sativa strain that has a medium (15–19%) amount of THC, with very little (<1%) CBD. It contains the terpene caryophyllene, which is useful in neve pain as well as depression.

Sour Dream is a sativa-predominant hybrid strain that has a medium (16–20%) amount of THC, with very little (<1%) CBD. It is a hybrid of two very popular cannabis strains, Blue Dream and Sour Diesel. It has myrcene as its predominant terpene, which can help with relaxation.

Ultimate Train Wreck is another sativa-predominant hybrid strain with a variable amount of THC, depending on where it is grown, but usually in the medium (15%) range.

Atomic Northern Lights is an indica-leaning hybrid with a low-to-medium (14%) amount of THC, with very little (<1%) CBD. Limonene and alpha-Pinene are its primary terpenes, so an uplifting mood as well as pain relief are typical properties, despite it being indica predominant, and like other strains for sexual dysfunction, it contains some myrcene.

Hindu Skunk is another indica-predominant hybrid, but with a higher amount (22%) of THC, with very little (<1%) CBD. It has caryophyllene as its main terpene, which is considered cannabinoidlike because it has a strong affinity for the CB2 receptors and thus can help with inflammation and nerve pain. Myrcene is also a prevalent terpene for relaxation.

Granddaddy Purple (GDP) is a pure indica that has a medium (15–19%) amount of THC, with very little (<1%) CBD. Like some of the other strains in this list, GDP has myrcene and caryophyllene as its terpenes and can be useful for female sexual disorders for its relaxing and sedating properties.

CBD for Female Sexual Disorders

CBD is the nonpsychoactive cannabinoid in medical cannabis and is also found in hemp. While combinations of both THC and CBD can be effective for a variety of conditions, including sexual dysfunction, there is much less evidence that CBD alone can be helpful to treat female sexual disorders. However, there are several reasons that CBD by itself may be effective. As previously mentioned, many female sexual disorders can be associated with anxiety, and there is evidence that CBD is effective for general anxiety. While there are a few small studies that show that high-dose CBD might reduce acute anxiety before a stressful event, such as public speaking,[6] CBD has better evidence if taken on a daily basis, at lower doses (around 25 mg daily), to reduce general anxiety.[7] Another reason why CBD may be effective in female sexual disorders is related to blood flow. Like THC, there is some extremely limited data that (at least in rats) CBD may dilate blood vessels,[8] which is certainly important to achieving and maintaining an erection in men and may have an important role in female sexual function as well.

While you can either use cannabis-derived CBD or hemp-derived CBD for daily treatment of anxiety, I generally recommend hemp-derived CBD because it is usually less expensive, and you can obtain this without certification. However, because hemp-derived CBD is not regulated by the FDA, you must be very careful that you are getting a high-quality, full-spectrum, third-party-verified product. For the treatment of female sexual disorders, I recommend 25 to 30 mg of CBD a day, which can be obtained by using CBD oil/tincture under the tongue, or CBD oil capsules. CBD, in general, does not immediately alleviate sexual dysfunction, but rather taken daily for at least one to two weeks, it can start to affect some of the chemical signaling in the brain that contribute to normal sexual function. Thus, don't expect to see improvement in symptoms right away.

Using Different Formulations for Female Sexual Disorders

Almost as important as which strain of cannabis you use, or the ratio of THC to CBD, is the formulation you use for sexual dysfunction. This is because different formulations have different onset of actions and different durations. Most sexual issues occur "in the moment." Thus, a rapid onset of action (works in second or minutes) is likely going to be more effective. However, as mentioned, some sexual issues are due to conditions like stress or anxiety, which could be constantly present, and therefore best treated with something that lasts a long time.

Tinctures are liquids that come in droppers. You place drops of tincture under your tongue to allow for fast absorption, rather than swallowing them directly. Tinctures take about thirty minutes to work and last four to six hours. Tinctures are also generally easier to titrate (slowly adjust) the dose, since doses can be increased drop by drop. Tinctures are often available in a variety of ratios of CBD to THC, which allows for further customization of balancing improvement in sexual function with sedation or getting "high." In addition, while this varies state by state, though most tinctures are extractions of primarily THC and CBD, some tinctures are available in sativa, indica, or hybrid strains, and some states sell extracts of the whole cannabis plant, so you can use a specific strain, like the ones listed above.

Pills or capsules (edibles) take a bit longer to work (one to two hours), but last longer in the body (up to eight hours), so they can be an excellent choice for something that may be contributing to sexual dysfunction, like anxiety. However, unlike Viagra for men, this is not a pill you want to take prior to sexual activity, as it may take too long to start working. Depending on the state, some edibles may be available as an indica, sativa, or hybrid and may even be available in a specific strain.

Vape comes in the form of a concentrated liquid (called "**concentrate**") that is extracted from the marijuana plant, and usually heated so it can be inhaled. Vape also works very quickly (seconds to minutes), which is very beneficial in sexual disorders, as they often occur in the moment. However, it also doesn't last very long (an hour or so), meaning that any sedation or other effects will disappear quickly. Almost all cannabis strains come in vape or concentrate, so you can choose one of those listed above (or similar) to start with.

Suppositories are a formulation not previously mentioned in this book, as female medical issues are probably the one major application for this formulation and are not typically found in most dispensaries. Suppositories are somewhat like edibles in that they take some time to work, are long lasting, and can affect the entire body. However, they are also like topicals in that they can primarily affect the area they are applied to. Suppositories may be particularly useful for menstrual cramps, pain during intercourse (dyspareunia), and even endometriosis (a condition causing chronic pelvic pain). Cannabis used via a suppository may also help with vaginal lubrication and thus enhance the sexual experience. Foria Relief, available in California and Colorado, makes a suppository that, according to one website, contains "a specially formulated blend of THC and CBD, cannabinoids which are known to relax muscles and release tension and cramping in the body[9]."

Oils and lubricants are other formulations not previously mentioned in this book, again because female medical issues are probably the one major application for these formulations, and they are also not typically found in most dispensaries. They are essentially topical formulations, but are primarily designed to be used during intercourse. Whether or not oils and other lubricants infused with cannabinoids can be helpful for female sexual disorders is unclear. However, they might help and are unlikely to be harmful. Curio Wellness offers aromatic intimacy oil infused with THC.

General Recommendations for Using Medical Cannabis and CBD in Women with Sexual Disorders

Because female sexual disorders and their causes can be very different (decreased sexual drive is very different from pain during intercourse, which is very different from the inability to have an orgasm), the best way to think about using medical cannabis and CBD for female sexual disorders is to try to consider all of the factors involved and then select the appropriate cannabis treatment based on how the strain and/or formulation works to help with these issues. Finally, different people react differently to different strains and formulations of cannabis. In general, I recommend a "start low, go slow" approach, and the same is true for sexual disorders. Thus, it might take some time to find the right strain and right formulation to treat your sexual dysfunction, so patience is warranted.

1. **In general, start by using a vape fifteen to twenty minutes before anticipated sexual activity.**

    Vape is probably the best formulation for sexual dysfunction in women. It can be taken before sexual activity to help with a variety of issues related to sexual dysfunction in women. While everyone reacts differently to different strains, I would start with an indica-leaning hybrid like **Atomic Northern Lights** or **Hindu Skunk**, though many women find they prefer sativa strains or sativa hybrids. If vape is not preferred, tincture is also a good option, though since it takes a bit longer to work, you need to take it at least thirty minutes before sexual activity. Since the first strain or formulation you try may not work, don't give up. Finding the right cannabis treatment often takes some trial and error, and this is especially true for female sexual disorders.

2. **Use daily CBD edibles (or tincture) if you have anxiety or stress that may be playing a role in your sexual dysfunction.** Again, it is unclear whether or not CBD alone can help with sexual issues in women. However, since we know it helps in anxiety, women who believe anxiety is a component of their sexual dysfunction should consider daily CBD. CBD may also decrease inflammation and increase blood flow, which can both be contributing factors certain causes of sexual dysfunction in women. I recommend 25 mg to 30 mg of CBD a day in a pill/edible/capsule or tincture. This can either be a marijuana-derived CBD or pure-hemp-derived CBD, though I generally recommend hemp-derived CBD, as it is less expensive and easier to obtain, and because there is virtually no THC, it will not make you sleepy or high.

3. **Consider suppositories, oils, and lubricants if pain and dryness are factors and if they are available in your area.** Unfortunately, cannabinoids containing suppositories, oils, and lubricants are not available in most areas. In addition, there is limited experience with these products and no research. Based on their mechanism of action, these are probably best used where pain and dryness is a significant factor in sexual dysfunction. Since the genitals are particularly sensitive areas with a lot of blood vessels that can absorb these products, start first with a very small amount (a tiny bit of oil, a quarter of a suppository) not before sexual activity, just to determine if your body reacts well to the product. If there are no adverse reactions, then a regular dose can be applied before sexual activity. If these products are not available in your area, there are hemp-based CBD products (Foria is one example) that can be purchased online, though the efficacy of these products are less clear.

4. Consider nonpharmacological approaches to sexual dysfunction.

Sexual disorders are complex, and since pharmaceuticals are limited, many nonpharmacologic options have been and continue to be used successfully today. There are various forms of counseling and behavior approaches that have helped many women with sexual disorders. While beyond the scope of this book, there are many therapists and other professionals who are experts in this area.

Chapter 26 Notes

1. Wiebe, E., and A. Just. How Cannabis Alters Sexual Experience: A Survey of Men and Women. *J Sex Med* 2019: 16, 1758–1762.

2. Sun, A. J., M. L. Eisenberg. Association Between Marijuana Use and Sexual Frequency in the United States: A Population-Based Study. *J Sex Med* 2017: 14, 1342–1347.

3. Wei, D., D. Lee, C. D. Cox, et al. Endocannabinoid signaling mediates oxytocin-driven social reward. *PNAS* November 10, 2015: 112(45), 14084–14089.

4. Ellis, E. F., S. F. Moore, and K. A. Willoughby. Anandamide and delta 9-THC dilation of cerebral arterioles is blocked by indomethacin. *Am J Physiol Heart Circ Physiol* 1995: 269, H1859–64.

5. Lynn, B. K., J. D. Lopez, C. Miller, et al. The relationship between marijuana use prior to sex and sexual function in women. *Sex Med* 2019: 7, 192–197.

6. Bergamaschi, M. M., R. H. Queiroz, et al. Cannabidiol reduces the anxiety induced by simulated public speaking in treatment-naïve social phobia patients. *Neuropsychopharmacology* 2011 May: 36(6), 1219–26.

7. Shannon, S., et al. Cannabidiol in Anxiety and Sleep: A Large Case Series. *Perm J* 2019: 23, 18–041.

8. Offertaler, L., F. M. Mo, S. Bátkai, et al. Selective ligands and cellular effectors of a G protein-coupled endothelial cannabinoid receptor. *Mol Pharmacol* 2003: 63, 699–705.

9. https://greendragon.com/product/foria/. Accessed 7/28/2020.

Chapter 27:

How to Use Medical Cannabis and CBD in Fibromyalgia, Chronic Fatigue, and Other Complex Medical Conditions

Complex Medical Conditions

While the other chapters in this section are the conditions I commonly see when certifying patients for medical cannabis, many of the patients I see for cannabis certification fall into a category I would like to call "complex medical conditions." While medical conditions can all be complex, there are certain conditions that patients face that can be particularly challenging because the cause of the condition is not well understood, or treatment options are limited. Some complex medical conditions have names like *fibromyalgia* or *chronic fatigue syndrome*. However, some conditions patients have are incredibly unique to that particular patient. These conditions are also complex because while their causes are not well understood, there are usually multiple factors such as stress, diet, and activity that can play important roles. Stress and anxiety are often a double-edged sword, because while there are effective treatments for stress and anxiety, these treatments alone are often not effective for these conditions, and many doctors will dismiss patients with complex medical conditions, thinking, "It's all in their head." Complex medical conditions often come together (e.g., fibromyalgia and chronic fatigue) or usually occur with other medical conditions (e.g., migraine and chronic fatigue), making the situation even more complex. While all complex medical conditions can be different in every patient, in my experience there tend to be three issues that seem to connect all of these conditions: inflammation, neuropathic pain, and stress.

Inflammation is the body's natural healing process. When something gets injured or infected, the body starts a cascade of activity known as inflammation that fights infection, begins healing, and even wards off cancer. When you catch a cold and get a fever and runny nose, or when you sprain an ankle and get pain and swelling, that's inflammation. One of the consequences of inflammation is pain, which can actually be protective. Pain is telling your body to rest or not use your sprained ankle. However, chronically, inflammation can cause many problems, including pain. A very common type of chronic pain is caused by inflammation is arthritis. However, chronic inflammation throughout the body can cause a variety of adverse effects.

Neuropathic pain is pain caused by damaged nerves. The most common type of neuropathic pain is diabetic neuropathic pain, also called diabetic neuropathy. A combination of elevated blood sugar and impaired circulation causes damage to nerves, most commonly in the lower extremities. However, there are other things that can damage nerves (infection, trauma, diseases of the nerves) and cause neuropathic pain. When nerves are damaged, they send incorrect signals, some of which are perceived as pain. Neuropathic pain is often described as burning or electric, but it can also cause numbness and weakness.

Stress can affect all medical conditions, but those with complex medical conditions tend to be even more affected by stress. The stress response is an evolutionary development that protected humans from predators and environmental stressors. However, that same stress response can kick in during mental stress, and if chronic, it can lead to a host of medical problems. It is very likely that patients with complex medical conditions, especially those where pain is involved, have genetic predisposition to increased sensitivity and pain during stress or periods of anxiety.

Medical Cannabis for Complex Medical Conditions

Fortunately, medical cannabis is an excellent option for patients with complex medical conditions for a variety of reasons. First, as mentioned, inflammation, neuropathic pain, and stress play an important role in many complex medical conditions, and medical cannabis and CBD can help with all three of these simultaneously. We know that medical cannabis can reduce pain,[1, 2, 3] decrease anxiety,[4, 5, 6] and at least CBD can decrease inflammation.[7, 8] Second, unlike typical medical conditions, pharmaceutical options for patients with complex medical conditions are typically quite limited and often do not work. Thus, medical cannabis presents a viable option. Finally, as mentioned, complex medical conditions often come together, or usually occur with other more typical medical conditions, and medical cannabis and CBD can treat a multitude of medical conditions simultaneously.

Strains for Complex Medical Conditions

Cannabis contains many different substances (called cannabinoids) that have medicinal properties. In addition to THC (the component that can make you "high") and CBD (which does not make you high), there are substances called terpenes that give cannabis its smell and flavor. The combination and proportion of cannabinoids and terpenes will help determine which strains are best to treat your condition . In generally, there are no randomized studies that have compared the various strains of cannabis plants and have determined which is the most effective for specific medical conditions. Thus, it can be challenging for people with less common and more complex conditions to choose the appropriate cannabis strain. Sativa strains are more uplifting, and indica strains tend to be more sedating and relaxing. However, depending on the situation and the patient, indica, sativa, or a hybrid of the two might work better. The terpene profile of a particular strain may be even more important than whether a strain is sativa or indica.

Two terpenes that can be beneficial for many complex conditions are beta-caryophyllene and myrcene. Beta-caryophyllene has a black pepper taste and smell and is helpful for both nerve pain and inflammation. Myrcene, which can also be found in hops, mango, and lemongrass, has muscle-relaxation properties in addition to helping with both pain and inflammation. While at the end of this chapter, I have listed some strains that have been found to do well in specific complex medical conditions, one general recommendation for patients with complex medical conditions is to try a variety of "classic" or popular strains that are high in myrcene and caryophyllene. A few of these strains are listed below:

Sour Diesel, Jack Herer, and **Green Crack** are all sativa strains that have a medium (15–20%) amount of THC, with very little (<1%) CBD and can be useful in low doses for elderly patients. They appear to be particularly good as mood elevators in these patients who tend to have depressed moods. They also all have caryophyllene, which is anti-inflammatory and also helpful with nerve issues. Sour Diesel (and to a lesser degree Green Crack) is high in limonene, which is relaxing. Green Crack has myrcene, which can also be calming.

Blue Dream is a sativa-predominant hybrid strain that has a medium (16–20%) amount of THC, with very little (<1%) CBD. It has myrcene as its predominant terpene, which can help with relaxation.

White Widow is a hybrid strain that has about 20% THC and 1% CBD that works well for all types of pain and can improve mood and cause relaxation.

ACDC is another balanced hybrid strain that is helpful for pain but is known for its low levels of THC. It has the opposite ratio of White Widow, with a 20:1 CBD-to-THC ratio. Thus, this is one strain that will not make you high. Its predominant terpene is beta-myrcene, which can be helpful for pain.

Blue Cheese is an indica-predominant (80%) hybrid strain. It also has a medium (14–18%) amount of THC, and very little (<1%) CBD. While it has caryophyllene and some myrcene like GDP and Northern Lights, its primary terpene is limonene. This, as well as the small sativa component, gives it a tiny bit of uplifting feeling, and thus it can be used in insomnia associated with anxiety and depression.

Granddaddy Purple (GDP) is a pure indica that has a medium (15–19%) amount of THC, with very little (<1%) CBD. GDP has myrcene and caryophyllene as its terpenes and can be useful in both anxiety and insomnia, which can be seen in patients with cancer.

Northern Lights is another pure indica, like GDP, with a medium (14–19%) amount of THC, and very little (<1%) CBD. Its predominant terpenes are myrcene and caryophyllene. Like GDP, it is also useful for insomnia and anxiety, which is seen in cancer. In addition, Northern Lights can be useful in nausea.

CBD for Complex Medical Conditions

While THC, the psychoactive component of medical cannabis, is extremely effective for pain, CBD is the nonpsychoactive component of cannabis that can be effective by itself, particularly for two aspects of complex medical conditions: inflammation and anxiety. As mentioned, CBD has been shown to have some anti-inflammatory properties.[7, 8] In terms of anxiety, there are a few small studies that show that high-dose CBD might reduce acute anxiety before a stressful event, such as public speaking.[9] CBD has better evidence if taken on a daily basis, at lower doses (around 25 mg daily) to reduce general anxiety.[10] Another property of CBD is that it has been found in mostly nonhuman studies to be neuroprotective, which means that it has been shown to help lessen the damage of brain and other nerve cells affected by conditions such as stroke, including the possibility of helping the growth of new brain cells,[11] so it may be particularly helpful in complex medical conditions where neuropathic pain is an important factor.

While you can use both marijuana-derived CBD or hemp-derived CBD for pain and inflammation, I recommend hemp-derived CBD because it is generally less expensive and you can obtain this without certification. However, because hemp-derived CBD is not regulated by the FDA, you must be very careful that you are getting a high-quality, full-spectrum, third-party-verified product. For almost all complex medical conditions, I recommend 25 to 30 mg of CBD a day, which can be obtained by using CBD oil/tincture under the tongue, or CBD oil capsules.

Using Different Formulations for Complex Medical Conditions

Almost as important as which strain of cannabis you use, or the ratio of THC to CBD, are the formulations used for complex medical conditions. This is because different formulations have different onsets of actions and different durations. Acute or severe pain requires a rapid onset of action (works in second or minutes), while chronic daily issues are best treated with something that lasts a long time. Patients with complex medical conditions, especially when pain is involved, usually have a combination of both things (e.g., acute and chronic pain). Thus, most patients with complex medical conditions will need to use both a variety of strains and a variety of formulations.

Tinctures are liquids that come in droppers. You place drops of tincture under your tongue to allow for fast absorption, rather than swallowing them directly. Tinctures take about thirty minutes to work and last four to six hours. Tinctures are also generally easier to titrate (slowly adjust) the dose, since doses can be increased drop by drop. Tinctures are often available in a variety of ratios of CBD to THC, which allows for further customization of balancing pain relief and sedation or getting "high." In addition, while this varies state by state, though most tinctures are extractions of primarily THC and CBD, some tinctures are available in sativa, indica, or hybrid strains, and some states sell extracts of the whole cannabis plant, so you can use a specific strain, like the ones listed above or below.

Pills or capsules (edibles) take a bit longer to work (one to two hours) but last longer in the body (up to eight hours). Since most complex medical conditions are constantly there, edibles are usually part of a cannabis regimen for patients, including CBD products. However, edibles are not good for symptoms that come on suddenly, like acute pain, as it may take too long to start working. Depending on the state, some edibles may be available as an indica, sativa, or hybrid and may even be available in a specific strain.

Vape comes in the form of a concentrated liquid (called "**concentrate**") that is extracted from the marijuana plant, and usually heated so it can be inhaled. Vape also works very quickly (seconds to minutes), which is very beneficial for symptoms that come on suddenly, such as acute pain. However, vape also doesn't last very long (an hour or so), meaning that any sedation or other effects will disappear quickly. Almost all cannabis strains come in vape or concentrate, so you can choose one of those listed above (or similar) to start with.

Topical formulations of medical cannabis come in salves and balms and can be highly effective for local pain. Despite having a high amount of THC, because they are applied to the skin, very little is absorbed in the bloodstream, and thus topical formulations have no psychoactive properties. Balms or creams only last a few hours and thus should be applied regularly. They are particularly good for pain, but usually only when it occurs on a specific area of the body, such as low-back pain. One downside of topical formulations is that they tend to be much more expensive than other formulations. Spreading a topical over your entire body can be quite expensive, so I generally recommend topicals only for localized pain.

General Recommendations for Complex Medical Conditions

It is difficult to recommend a specific regimen in a handout or book even for a common medical problem because every patient's experience of the same problem can be so different, and every patient will react somewhat differently to the different strains, formulations, and amounts of THC. This is even more true for complex medical problems. However, below are some general principles that can be applied to most complex medical conditions, as well as some specific recommendations for a few common complex medical conditions that do not otherwise have a separate chapter in this book.

1. **Start low, go slow.**

   Please remember that since the general recommendation for using medical cannabis it to "start low, go slow," you will likely need some patience when using medical cannabis to treat pain, especially chronic pain.

2. **Take a daily, high-dose CBD capsule pill or tincture daily.**

   CBD has anti-inflammatory properties, which can reduce pain and inflammation seen in many complex chronic conditions. Thus, any patient with a complex medical condition should take CBD daily, not only to treat symptoms like pain but to also treat the cause of the symptom in a preventative manner. This is especially true for chronic pain from inflammation, such as osteoarthritis. CBD also has a salutary effect on neurotransmitters, which play an important role in many complex conditions. Start with 25 mg to 30 mg of CBD daily in either a pill/capsule or tincture. This can either be a cannabis-derived CBD or a full-spectrum hemp-derived CBD. I generally recommend hemp-derived CBD, as it is less expensive and easier to obtain, and because there is virtually no THC, it will not make you sleepy or high.

3. **For symptoms that are present on a regular basis, use edibles or tincture several times a day with low amounts of THC, usually in a 2:1 or 1:1 ratio of CBD to THC.**

   Patients with complex medical conditions, including pain syndromes, usually have a low level of their underlying condition that is always there, punctuated by episodes of increased symptoms. Thus, regular use of pills/edible or tinctures should help keep complex conditions under better control. This usually involves using edibles or tinctures about two to four times a day, depending on the other cannabis products you are taking, and whether you use edibles or tinctures. While edibles and tinctures come in a variety of ratios of CBD to THC (14:1, 4:1, 1:1, 1:4, et cetera), since I recommend that patients take higher doses of daily CBD, I have found it much easier (and less expensive) for patients to stick with 2:1 or 1:1 products, as above. Since pills and tinctures are often reconstituted with terpenes added back, choose products specifically designed for your specific conditions; for example, look for terpenes such as beta-caryophyllene and myrcene if pain is involved. While each state is different, some companies make edibles and tinctures that are either sativa, indica, or hybrid, and some companies even make strain-specific products, so you can use strains that others have found best for your conditions (several are listed below). Start with approximately 0.5 to 1 mg of THC for the first dose. You can figure out how much THC is in one pill or one dropperful of tincture by looking at the package. For example, a 2:1 tincture that comes in a 15-ml bottle with 300 mg cannabinoids, half a dropperful (0.5 ml or 10 drops) contains 10 mg of cannabinoids. So three drops will be about 2 mg of CBD and 1 mg THC. You can start with about five drops (1–2 mg of THC) each day, or even with each dose, and then slowly increase the amount of THC drop by drop until you get the desired amount of pain relief without side effects. Edibles are easier to dose because the milligrams are stated on the package, and you can usually easily cut an edible in half or quarter to achieve your desired dose. Most patients achieve good results at 2 to 10 mg of THC per dose.

4. **Use vape for severe and acute symptoms.**

As stated above, most patients with complex medical conditions have a constant low level of their underlying condition, punctuated by episodes of increased symptoms. Thus, when these acute symptoms arise, something that works quickly like vape is needed. Whereas CBD is taken every day, and pills and tincture mixes of THC and CBD are taken regularly several times a day, vape can be used for when pain flares up or is severe. Be sure to use a vape that is a concentrate from a cannabis strain that is particularly good for your condition or symptoms (some are listed below). Start with one puff at the onset of symptoms, and wait a few minutes to determine its effect. Slowly increase your dose by one puff at a time. Eventually, you will determine the number of puffs it takes to relieve acute symptoms without getting sleepy or high.

5. **For symptoms limited to a small area of the body (e.g., right shoulder) consider topical preparations.**
Topical balms and ointments can be very effective for patients with localized pain (i.e., pain in once specific area). It can either be used in addition to the regimen above or used exclusively for localized pain. Also, since many complex medical conditions have multiple areas of where pain is involved (e.g., fibromyalgia), topicals can be effective for the most troublesome spot. Unless the condition is related to the skin (psoriasis, eczema), I do not find CBD topicals particularly effective, so use high-concentration THC balms or ointments.

6. **Address any sleep-related issues.**
Patient with complex medical conditions, especially if pain is involved, will commonly have difficulty with sleep. Fortunately, cannabis is also very good at making people sleepy. In addition, to THC and CBD, there is also CBN, which stands for cannabinol. Like CBD, CBN is a nonpsychoactive cannabinoid, and CBN is particularly good for sleep. Five milligrams of CBN may be as effective as a 10-mg dose of diazepam (generic for Valium) for inducing sleep. There are both tinctures and edibles that come in 1:1 CBN:THC ratios. Some also contain natural ingredients such as chamomile and melatonin that can be quite effective to help induce sleep. In addition, some tinctures and edibles contain THC from indica strains, and in some states, you can get tinctures as a whole-plant extract of a particular strain. Since tinctures only take about twenty to thirty minutes to work and last about four to six hours, an indica-based tincture, especially one containing CBN, is often a great place to start as it can help patients both fall asleep and stay asleep. Start with ½ dropperful thirty minutes before bedtime and

increase by a ¼ to ½ dropperful each evening until you are falling asleep easily and staying asleep. For patients who have more issues staying asleep than falling asleep, a pill or edible may be a better option. While pills or edibles take about an hour to start working, they last six to eight hours. A 5-mg THC edible, particularly if an indica strain and/or contains CBN would be another good option. Start with a half tablet for the first night or two. If that doesn't work, then go up to the one full tablet. You can increase by half a tablet every two nights until you are staying asleep.

7. **Continue regular medicines (especially daily opioids and antidepressants) at least initially.**
Complex medical conditions are complex. While multiple forms of medical cannabis may effectively treat a complex medical condition where other more traditional treatments have failed, in my experience patients with complex medical conditions have had the best success when using medical cannabis in conjunction with their regular (usually prescription medication) treatments. This is especially true of opioids and antidepressants, the latter of which are commonly used for complex medical conditions to deal with neurotransmitter abnormalities. Stopping these medications quickly can lead to withdrawal and serious side effects. My goal for treating any patient, and especially those with complex medical conditions, is not to get them off all prescription medications (though that would be wonderful), but rather to control their symptoms in order to have an improved quality of life. Once symptoms are well controlled, then reducing prescription medications that may no longer be needed can be addressed. While certain medications (prescription sleeping medications like zolpidem, or anxiety medications like alprazolam) can be more easily replaced with cannabis substitutes, since medical cannabis and CBD tend to have complementary actions to prescription medications, often the best results are achieved by combining both medical cannabis/CBD with prescription medications.

Fibromyalgia

Fibromyalgia is a chronic condition that causes pain all over the body and affects about four million US adults, or 2% of the adult population.[12] Fibromyalgia patients also have problems with sleep and energy, and there is typically an association between symptoms and stress, anxiety, and/or depression. Like other syndromes, the cause of fibromyalgia is unknown, but there is some thought that patients with fibromyalgia are simply more sensitive to pain than most people.

Medical cannabis and CBD could play an important role in conditions such as fibromyalgia, as researchers have found that individuals affected with these conditions have low levels of endocannabinoids compared to those without these medical conditions.[13] This concept of endocannabinoid deficiency is changing our understanding of several related diseases that many doctors and researchers continue to believe are mostly psychosomatic. Unfortunately, the evidence for the use of medical cannabis and CBD in fibromyalgia is scant. One review of two studies of a synthetic cannabis product (not available in the United States) did not show any major improvement in fibromyalgia patients taking this product.[14] However, one survey of fibromyalgia patients found cannabis to be of benefit,[15] and another study using inhaled pharmaceutical-grade cannabis in twenty fibromyalgia patients found some pain relief.[16]

Recommendations: Since fibromyalgia is mostly a pain syndrome, the recommendations regarding pain in the previous chapter on chronic pain (Chapter 17) should mostly apply. While I recommend that most patients with chronic pain take CBD, since fibromyalgia may be related to endocannabinoid deficiency and CBD has evidence in treating neuropathic conditions, I would even more strongly recommend that patients with fibromyalgia take daily CBD at doses of 25 mg to 30 mg each day. In terms of strains, while I recommend the same strains for chronic pain (White Widow, Harlequin, Jack Flash, and ACDC) recommended in the chronic pain chapter, there are some additional strains that seem to work well in patients with fibromyalgia.

Cannatonic is a balanced hybrid, but like ACDC, has low (but slightly higher) amounts (3–7%) of THC, as well as medium amounts

(6–10%) of CBD, with myrcene as a predominant terpene. **Blue Dream** is a sativa-predominant hybrid strain that also has a medium (16–20%) amount of THC, with very little (<1%) CBD, and it has myrcene as its predominant terpene. **Girl Scout Cookies (GSC)** is a balanced hybrid, with a high-THC concentration and little CBD, which is used for severe pain.

Chronic Fatigue Syndrome

Chronic Fatigue Syndrome (CFS) is a chronic condition where patients feel tired all the time. It has also been called myalgic encephalomyelitis. While the cause of CFS is not known, the term *encephalomyelitis* means inflammation of the brain and spinal cord, and thus the term is used as many believe CFS is due to some sort of infection (viral, bacterial) or other inflammatory abnormality that leads to inflammation of the of the brain and/or spinal cord. Myalgias are muscle pains that can accompany CFS. In fact, there is a likely an overlap between CFS and fibromyalgia. In addition to having chronic fatigue, patients with CFS tend to have worse symptoms with increased activity, which can be incredibly debilitating. In addition to muscle pain and fatigue, CFS patients can also have issues with sleep. Somewhere between 836,000 to 2.5 million Americans suffer from CFS, though most of them have not been diagnosed.[17]

Like fibromyalgia, medical cannabis and CBD could play an important role in chronic fatigue syndrome, as researchers have found that affected individuals have low levels of endocannabinoids,[13] suggesting that chronic fatigue is actually caused by an endocannabinoid deficiency. In addition, since inflammation appears to be important in the development of the disease, medical cannabis and CBD in particular have anti-inflammatory properties. Unfortunately, there is currently only anecdotal evidence that medical cannabis and CBD can help with CFS.[18] However, three hallmarks of CFS can be treated successfully with medical cannabis: depression, insomnia, and muscle pain. Focusing on these symptoms should be effective for patients with CFS.

Recommendations: Since the predominant symptoms of CFS are depression, insomnia, and chronic pain, the recommendations from the previous chapters on these subjects (Chapter 15, Chapter 14, and Chapter 17, respectively), should be a good starting point, with the focus on the most bothersome symptom first. Similar to fibromyalgia, while I recommend that most patients with chronic pain take CBD, since CFS may be related to both and endocannabinoid deficiency and inflammation, and CBD has evidence of having anti-inflammatory properties, I would even more strongly recommend that patients with CFS take daily CBD at doses of 25 mg to 30 mg each day. In terms of strains, sativas and sativa-dominant hybrids, especially those with myrcene and limonene, can be quite effective. Thus, the first few strains listed in Chapter 15 for depression (Jack Herer, Green Crack, Blue Dream, OG Kush, and Harlequin) are excellent strains to start with. Granddaddy Purple (also in Chapter 15) is an indica strain that is excellent for sleep. In addition, another strain, **Durban Poison**, has been reported to be effective ins CFS patients. Durban Poison is a pure sativa strain that contains a medium (14–19%) amount of THC, with very little (<1%) CBD, and its predominant terpene is terpinolene followed by myrcene. Formulations will primarily be edible, though for acute pain or problems with insomnia, vape might be helpful.

Burning Mouth Syndrome

Burning mouth syndrome is a condition (and another syndrome) where patients get chronic pain, burning, or otherwise unpleasant sensation in their mouth. The cause is unknown, and it remains difficult to both diagnose and treat.[19] It can be associated with damage to the mouth (dental work) or other chemical exposures. Damage to nerves is thought to play a role, and burning mouth syndrome can be considered a form of neuropathy. There is a wide variety of agents that have been tried to treat burning mouth syndrome, including gabapentin and other prescription medications found to be effective in neuropathies. There may be an important role for medical cannabis and CBD in patients with burning mouth syndrome, as one study that biopsied the mouths of individuals with and without the condition found that patients with burning mouth syndrome had decreased CB1 receptors and increased CB2 receptors in the cells of their tongue that were located in the areas where symptoms occurred.[20]

Recommendations: Since burning mouth syndrome is quite uncommon, there are no specific strains or formulations that have been reported to be particularly beneficial in patients with this condition. Since this is a neuropathic condition, I would recommend taking daily CBD. In addition, I would recommend strains that contain myrcene and pinene, which are terpenes that are particularly good for pain. Tinctures may be a particularly good formulation for patients with burning mouth, as that application to the spot on the tongue that is symptomatic may have some local or topical effects as well.

Diabetic Peripheral Neuropathy

Diabetic peripheral neuropathy is a complication of diabetes that can have a significant impact on patients. Damages to the nerves in the hands and feet in diabetics can not only cause pain and/or a burning sensation, but also loss of sensation. This loss of sensation can lead to limb damage, and in fact, diabetic related peripheral neuropathy and vascular disease are the leading causes for leg amputation in the United States. Diabetic nerve damage is caused by a combination of elevated blood sugar and impaired circulation seen in these patients, most commonly in the lower extremities. When nerves are damaged, they send incorrect signals, some of which are perceived as pain.

There is evidence that medical cannabis can be helpful in neuropathic pain. In one small study of twenty-one patients who had surgical or trauma induced peripheral neuropathy, an herbal cannabis preparation compared to placebo significantly reduced pain intensity.[21] In another similarly designed small (sixteen-patient) study of patients with diabetic peripheral neuropathy, smoking cannabis compared to placebo similarly reduced pain from diabetic peripheral neuropathy.[22]

Recommendations: Since diabetic peripheral neuropathy is a neuropathic condition, I would recommend taking daily CBD. Two strains that have been mentioned as helpful in diabetic peripheral neuropathy are White Widow (above) and Jack Flash, an indica-leaning (55%) hybrid strain. It also has a medium (18%) amount of THC, and very little (<1%) CBD. Its predominant terpene is linalool, which has analgesic and anticonvulsant properties. In addition, I would recommend any strains that contain myrcene and pinene, which are terpenes that are particularly good for pain. As above, patients with diabetic neuropathy can use edibles or tinctures for daily pain and vape for acute pain. Topical preparations may help, especially if pain is located to just the bottoms of the feet.

Chapter 27 Notes

1. Whiting, P. F., R. F. Wolff, S. Deshpande, et al. Cannabinoids for Medical Use: A Systematic Review and Meta-analysis. *JAMA* 2015 Jun 23–30: 313(24), 2456–73.

2. Boehnke, K. F., E. Litinas, and D. J. Clauw. Medical Cannabis Use Is Associated With Decreased Opiate Medication Use in a Retrospective Cross-Sectional Survey of Patients With Chronic Pain. *J Pain* 2016 Jun: 17(6), 739–44.

3. Abrams, D. I., P. Couey, S. B. Shade, et al. Cannabinoid-opioid interaction in chronic pain. *Clin Pharmacol Ther* 2011 Dec: 90(6), 844–51.

4. Regelson, W., J. R. Butler, J. Schulz, T. Kirk, L. Peek, M. L. Green, and M. O. Zalis. Delta 9-THC as an effective antidepressant and appetite-stimulating agent in advanced cancer patients. In M. C. Braude & S. Szara (Eds.), *The Pharmacology of Marihuana* (pp. 763–776). New York: Raven Press, 1976.

5. Fabre, L. F., and D. McLendon. The efficacy and safety of nabilone (a synthetic cannabinoid) in the treatment of anxiety. *J Clin Pharmacol* 1981 Aug–Sep: 21(S1), 377S–382S.

6. Greer, G. R., C. S. Grob, and A. L. Halberstadt AL. PTSD symptom reports of patients evaluated for the New Mexico Medical Cannabis Program. *J Psychoactive Drugs* 2014 Jan–Mar: 46(1), 73–7.

7. Xiong, W., C. Tanxing, et al. Cannabinoids suppress inflammatory and neuropathic pain by targeting α3 glycine receptors. *J Exp Med* 2012 Jun 4: 209(6), 1121–1134.

8. Philpott, H. T., M. O'Brien, and J. J. McDougall. Attenuation of early phase inflammation by cannabidiol prevents pain and nerve damage in rat osteoarthritis. *Pain* 2017: 158(12), 2442–2451.

9. Bergamaschi, M. M., R. H. Queiroz, et al. Cannabidiol reduces the anxiety induced by simulated public speaking in treatment-naïve social phobia patients. *Neuropsychopharmacology* 2011 May: 36(6), 1219–26.

10. Shannon, S., et al. Cannabidiol in Anxiety and Sleep: A Large Case Series. *Perm J* 2019: 23, 18–041.

11. Campos, A. C., M. V. Fogaça, A. B. Sonego, and F. S. Guimarães. Cannabidiol, neuroprotection and neuropsychiatric disorders. *Pharmacol Res* 2016 Oct: 112, 119–127.

12. Fibromyalgia. https://www.cdc.gov/arthritis/basics/fibromyalgia.htm accessed 5/21/20.

13. Russo, Ethan B. Clinical endocannabinoid deficiency reconsidered: current research supports the theory in migraine, fibromyalgia, irritable bowel, and other treatment-resistant syndromes. *Cannabis and cannabinoid research* 2016: 1(1), 154–165.

14. Walitt, B., P. Klose, M. A. Fitzcharles, T. Phillips, and W. Häuser. Cannabinoids for fibromyalgia. *Cochrane Database of Systematic Reviews* 2016: 7. Art. No.: CD011694. DOI: 10.1002/14651858. CD011694.pub2.

15. Fiz, J., M. Durán, D. Capellà, et al. Cannabis Use in Patients with Fibromyalgia: Effect on Symptoms Relief and Health-Related Quality of Life. *PLOS* 2011, April 21. https://doi.org/10.1371/journal. pone.0018440.

16. van de Donk, T., M. Niesters, M. A. Kowal, et al. An experimental randomized study on the analgesic effects of pharmaceutical-grade cannabis in chronic pain patients with fibromyalgia. *Pain* 2019: 160, 860–869.

17. Myalgic encephalomyelitis/chronic fatigue syndrome. https://www. cdc.gov/me-cfs/index.html. Accessed 5/22/2020.

18. Rowe, P. C., R. A. Underhill, K. J. Friedman, et al. Myalgic Encephalomyelitis/Chronic Fatigue Syndrome Diagnosis and Management in Young People: A Primer. *Front Pediatr* 2017: 5, 121.

19. Grushka, M., and N. Su. Burning Mouth Syndrome in João, NAR, Ferreira, J. F. (Ed.), *Orofacial Disorders: Current Therapies in Orofacial Pain and Oral Medicine* (pp. 223–232). 2017.

20. Borsani, E., A. Majorana, M. A. Cocchi, et al. Epithelial Expression of Vanilloid and Cannabinoid Receptors: A Potential Role in Burning Mouth Syndrome Pathogenesis. *Histol Histopathol* 2014 Apr: 29(4), 523–33.

21. Ware, M. A., T. Wang, S. Shapiro, et al. Smoked cannabis for chronic neuropathic pain: a randomized controlled trial. *CMAJ* 2010 Oct 5: 182(14), E694–E701.

22. Wallace, M. S., T. D. Marcotte, A. Umlauf, et al. Efficacy of Inhaled Cannabis on Painful Diabetic Neuropathy. *J Pain* 2015 Jul: 16(7), 616–627.

Chapter 28:

Treating the Elderly with Medical Cannabis and CBD

Why Consider Medical Cannabis and CBD in the Elderly

Perhaps the biggest reason for my interest in medical cannabis and CBD was its usefulness and underutilization in the geriatric population. As a primary care physician, I treat a variety of conditions, including diabetes, high cholesterol, high blood pressure, and emphysema—in all of which, the use of cannabis has an almost nonexistent role. While I do recommend medical cannabis to my regular patients where appropriate, most of the patients I see for medical cannabis certification have their own primary care physician, but he or she refuses or is unable to certify them for medical cannabis. Initially, these were the first patients I saw for medical cannabis certification, and in general, they were slightly younger than my regular primary care patients, most of whom are sixty-five and older. After successfully treating younger patients for conditions like pain, anxiety, and insomnia—all of which are extremely common in geriatric medicine—it one day dawned on me: "Why should I prescribe Ambien for one of my older patients, when cannabis is at least as effective and much safer?" As we get older, our bodies start to break down, and we tend to develop more and more chronic conditions. The current medical approach to the aging process seems to be prescribing additional medications. While I am not opposed to prescriptions, they come with side effects and interactions, which are compounded with each pill that is added—a condition known as polypharmacy, which is, not surprisingly, quite common in the elderly. The two main benefits of plant-based medicine, such as medical cannabis and CBD, are that they can treat a variety of conditions simultaneously, and with few side effects and interactions.

While medical cannabis is by no means an antiaging treatment or "fountain of youth," there is some evidence that it might be able to delay some of the damage caused by aging. The best examples of this are neuroprotection and joint inflammation. As we get older, there is naturally occurring damage to the brain and nerve cells. Cannabidiol (CBD) has been found in mostly nonhuman studies to be neuroprotective, which means that it has been shown to help lessen the effects of damaged brain cells in conditions such as stroke, including the possibility of helping the growth of new brain cells.[1] In addition to CBD, another cannabinoid found in cannabis, Δ9-tetrahydrocannabivarin, or THCV, was, at least in animal research models for Parkinson's disease, found to not only have neuroprotective effects, but also to relieve symptoms.[2] Inflammation is the body's natural healing process. When something gets injured or infected, the body starts a cascade of activity known as inflammation that fights infection, begins healing, and even wards off cancer. Osteoarthritis (OA) is the wear and tear of bones that everyone gets over time as a result of aging, and it is common in the elderly. Research has shown CBD may have direct effects on inflammatory cells or may modulate the effects of certain pain receptors in the spinal cord.[3] While human studies are lacking, in an experimental model using rats, CBD has been shown to prevent pain caused by joint inflammation.[4]

Unfortunately, medical cannabis and CBD is likely highly underutilized by the geriatric population, the reasons of which are multifactorial. Lack of education, of both patients and their physicians, is likely a major factor (and one of the reasons I have written this book). Stigma is likely another factor. While there is substantial variation among patients when it comes to the acceptance of using medical cannabis and CBD, I have found in my experience that younger seniors (those in their sixties and seventies) are more accepting since they were teens and young adults in the 1960s, when recreational marijuana use had a substantial increase, and older seniors (those in their eighties and nineties) are less comfortable, as they were the parents of those teenagers who were disapproving of this behavior.

Another likely significant factor is a concern for safety. Seniors are on multiple medications, as discussed, so the safety of cannabis interacting with other medications is a concern. In addition, seniors are more susceptible to adverse effects from any substance; thus side effects of cannabis are further potential safety concerns. Fortunately, medical cannabis is generally very safe and has few interactions with medications, thus making it a perfect choice for seniors. While there is extremely limited research using medical cannabis in the elderly, one study examining nearly three thousand seniors showed that not only was medical cannabis effective (97% of patients reported improvements in their condition), but there were also very few side effects, with the most common being dizziness (9.7%), dry mouth (7.1%), somnolence (3.9%), weakness (2.3%), and nausea (2.2%).[5] While dizziness is certainly a concern, as falls in the elderly can be serious, another study that observed 204 seniors seventy-five years and older found no increased risk of falls.[6] Given the potential benefit of helping with several common ailments of elderly patients, the ability of whole-plant medicines to reduce the number of prescriptions needed, the low risk of adverse reactions seen in a relatively large study, and limited interactions with other medications, the use of medical cannabis in the elderly has a huge potential for benefit in this patient population.

Treating Medical Conditions in the Elderly with Medical Cannabis and CBD

The elderly have many common and chronic medical conditions, of which many have a potential role for use of medical cannabis and CBD. In fact, almost all the proceeding chapters in this section of the book can be applied to the elderly. While the benefit of using medical cannabis and CBD in the elderly should now be clear, the complexity of using medical cannabis in the elderly has to do with treating multiple conditions simultaneously and using appropriate dosing and formulations for this population. The following are just a few of the many relevant conditions to consider when treating the elderly:

Dementia, as well as Alzheimer's disease, can be seen in the elderly. In addition, there are natural changes in the brain that do not amount to dementia but can be troubling for the elderly. In true dementia and Alzheimer's disease, neuropsychiatric symptoms can occur and include agitation, aggression, wandering, apathy, sleep disorders, depression, anxiety, psychosis, and eating disorders,[7] and research demonstrates that medical cannabis can help treat these conditions.[8]

Agitation and anxiety are both common in the elderly, including those with and without dementia. The role for medical cannabis and CBD in anxiety is well established. While high doses of THC can cause anxiety, low doses of THC can be calming, and CBD alone has robust evidence for treating anxiety.[9] Severe agitation in patients with dementia is often treated by using antipsychotic medications, which have serious side effects, including excessive drowsiness, rigidity, and unusual movements and have been linked to a higher risk of death for patients with dementia. Medical cannabis, especially low-dose THC, can be calming and help with both anxiety and agitation, without some of the serious adverse effects seen in prescription medications, especially the more serious side effects seen in antipsychotics.

Appetite: While also common in dementia, some older patients lose their appetite. This can be caused by a variety of reasons, including physiologic changes in taste, changes in environment, and even side effects from prescription medications.[10] Losing weight can predispose elderly patients to other medical conditions, and lack of proper nutrition can worsen dementia and other symptoms. The THC found in medical cannabis is known to stimulate appetite and can help prevent wasting.

Pain/Arthritis: Elderly patients generally have several chronic conditions, one of which is often chronic pain secondary to osteoarthritis. Osteoarthritis is the wear and tear of bones caused by overuse and aging. This process leads to inflammation, which causes pain. Chronic pain can be particularly tricky to manage in elderly patients, especially patients with dementia, as they may not be easily able to verbalize their pain symptoms. THC is quite good at alleviating pain directly, and the anti-inflammatory properties of CBD can decrease the inflammation that leads to chronic joint pain from osteoarthritis.

Insomnia: Insomnia is very common in elderly patients and stems from a variety of factors, including stress (recent death of a spouse), environmental factors (moving to an unfamiliar location), and biological factors such as changes in the sleep-wake cycle that occur with the aging process.[11] Fortunately, the cannabinoids, THC and CBN in particular, are effective at treating insomnia. The are many formulations, such as edibles and tinctures in most states where medical cannabis is legal, that have easy to administer medical cannabis products specifically designed for sleep. Since lack of sleep can affect so many other conditions, dealing with insomnia in the elderly is usually the first thing that should be addressed.

Strains for the Elderly

Cannabis contains many different substances (called cannabinoids) that have medicinal properties. In addition to THC (the component that can make you "high") and CBD (which does not make you high), there are substances called terpenes that give marijuana its smell and flavor. The combination and proportion of cannabinoids and terpenes determine the effects that cannabis has on the body, with different strains of the cannabis plant having different proportions of these substances and therefore different effects. The most common way of classifying different strains is dividing them into two categories: indica and sativa. Sativa strains are generally uplifting and energizing, while indica strains are generally more relaxing and sedating. Pinene is a common terpene that is typically found in most sativa strains and can be good for memory, and it is a good mood lifter, which can be helpful for elderly patients. Limonene and myrcene are also good terpenes for the elderly, as they can be relaxing and help with anxiety and sleep. Beta-caryophyllene is good for both inflammation and pain. There are also hybrid strains, which can be balanced (half indica/half sativa) or more predominant in one or the other. One of the complexities of treating elderly patients is that they have a variety of different symptoms. This can be solved by using a variety of strains and/or hybrid strains that can address multiple problems. Sativa or sativa-predominant hybrid strains can be useful in elderly patients during the day, because they are less sedating and are especially good for being both uplifting and calming. Indica or indica-predominant hybrids may be more useful for insomnia, acute pain, and acute agitation. For multiple issues at once, pure hybrids with several predominant terpenes may be quite effective. Finally, since seniors can be particularly sensitive to THC, having some low THC strains should be considered, especially when first starting out. While the various strains and terpenes can be effective in elderly patients to treat a variety of conditions, every patient is different, so it may take some trial and error to determine which strain is the right strain for you or your affected loved one. A few strains that elderly patients should consider have successfully used for a variety of common conditions include the following:

Sour Diesel, **Jack Herer**, and **Green Crack**. These are all sativa strains that have a medium (15–20%) amount of THC, with very little (<1%) CBD and can be useful in low doses for elderly patients. They appear to be particularly good as mood elevators in these patients who tend to have depressed moods. They also all have caryophyllene, which is anti-inflammatory and also helpful with nerve issues. Sour Diesel (and to a lesser degree Green Crack) is high in limonene, which is relaxing. Green Crack has myrcene, which can also be calming.

Blue Dream is a sativa-predominant hybrid strains that has a medium (16–20%) amount of THC, with very little (<1%) CBD. Myrcene is its predominant terpene, so it is good for relaxation, and also has pinene which is good for memory.

Harlequin is also a sativa-dominant hybrid, but with a much higher CBD-to-THC ratio (about 5:2). It has low amounts (3–6%) of THC and medium amounts (7–10%) of CBD. Harlequin is high in myrcene as well, and along with Green Crack, it is helpful for chronic fatigue. Because of its low THC, it can be an excellent strain to start with.

ACDC is also a balance hybrid strain, which can be helpful for both pain and anxiety. However, its known for having low levels of THC, with a 20:1 CBD-to-THC ratio. Thus, this is one strain that should not make you "high," and therefore is a great option to start with in the elderly.

Cannatonic is a also balanced hybrid, and like ACDC, has low (but slightly higher) amounts (3–7%) of THC, as well as medium amounts (6–10%) of CBD, with myrcene as a predominant terpene, so it is good for relaxation.

Granddaddy Purple (GDP) and **Northern Lights** are both pure indica strains with a medium (14–19%) amount of THC, with very little (<1%) CBD. Both have myrcene and caryophyllene as their predominant terpenes, so they are both useful in anxiety and insomnia associated with depression. Northern Lights also has a bit of limonene, so it can be a relaxing, sleep-inducing strain, that can simultaneously elevate mood.

CBD for the Elderly

CBD is the nonpsychoactive cannabinoid in medical cannabis and is also found in hemp. While it may have a role in dementia and similar neurologic issues due to neuroprotective effects,[1] it can be highly effective for both anxiety and inflammation. Thus, because of the many potential benefits of CBD in the elderly, lack of psychoactive effects, and general safety, CBD should likely be a part of any treatment plan for elderly patients. CBD has an additional benefit in that it appears to counterbalance some of the unwanted effects (sedation, feeling "high") that are associated with THC. While all cannabis strains contain both THC and CBD, some of the strains recommended for elderly patients may have high levels of THC with low levels of CBD. Thus, using CBD combined with high-THC strains that are recommend may be effective in helping with some of these unwanted effects of those strains.

While CBD-only products can be derived from either marijuana or hemp, I generally recommend hemp-derived CBD because it is usually less expensive, and you can obtain this without certification.

However, because hemp-derived CBD is not regulated by the FDA, you must be very careful that you are getting a high-quality, full-spectrum, third-party-verified product.

For most elderly patients, I recommend 25 mg to 30 mg of CBD a day, which can be ingested by using CBD oil/tincture under the tongue, or CBD oil capsules. One exception is that CBD can be an appetite suppressant, so elderly patients with appetite issues should use a lower amount (15mg or less) of CBD. CBD, in general, does not immediately alleviate anxiety, pain, depression, or other symptoms, but rather taken daily for at least one to two weeks, it can start to affect some of the chemical signaling in the brain and joints to take effect. Patients and caregivers should not expect to see improvement in patients' symptoms right away.

Using Different Formulations in the Elderly

Almost as important as which strain of cannabis you use, or things like the ratio of THC to CBD, is the formulation you use, particularly important when treating elderly patients. Some of this is due to the fact that different formulations have different onsets of actions and different durations. Certain symptoms, like chronic pain from inflammation or general anxiety, can be constant and require a long-acting agent, while severe pain or agitation can come on quickly and require a more rapid-acting agent. In addition, elderly patients—particularly those with dementia and arthritis—may have difficulty with certain formulations, such as those that require following a specific set of instructions and/or manual dexterity that must be followed on order to be used correctly.

Pills or capsules (edibles) take longer to work (about an hour hour), but last longer in the body (up to eight hours). Thus, edibles are great options for elderly patients with constant symptoms such as pain due to arthritis, depression, or generalized anxiety. Edibles are preferred in elderly patients both for their long-acting effects and ease of delivery. However, because they last longer, if the dose is too high, any adverse effects will also last longer, so caution with dosing in the elderly is highly recommended.

Tinctures are liquids that come in droppers. You place drops of tincture under your tongue to allow for fast absorption, rather than swallowing them directly. Tinctures take about thirty minutes to work and last four to six hours. There are two advantages to using tinctures in elderly patients. The first is that they are generally easier to titrate (slowly adjust) the dose, since doses can be increased drop by drop. This is particularly important for elderly patients, as doses should be started very low and slowly increased to prevent side effects. Secondly, tinctures may also be easier for caregivers to administer, which is especially important for elderly patients who may have dementia or who may not be able to swallow edibles and/or may not be appropriate for vaping. Finally, while this varies state by state, while most tinctures are extractions of primarily THC and CBD, some tinctures are available in sativa, indica, or hybrid strains, and some states sell extracts of the whole cannabis plant, so you can use a specific strain, like the ones listed above.

Vape commonly comes in the form of a concentrated liquid (called "**concentrate**") that is extracted from the cannabis plant, and usually heated so it can be inhaled. Vape also works very quickly (in seconds to minutes), which is greatly beneficial for acute and severe symptoms. However, it also does not last very long (an hour or so), meaning that vape alone is probably not practical for a condition that is always present, like general anxiety or pain from arthritis. In addition, vape requires following instructions and some coordination, which may not be possible for certain elderly patients. Thus, vape may not be the best options for all elderly patients. Where vape may be effective is for sudden and severe symptoms, such as acute pain or severe agitation, for patients who are able to follow instructions and coordinate breathing. Almost all cannabis strains come in vape or concentrate, so you can choose one of those listed above (or similar) to start with.

Topical agents can be used to deliver medical cannabis. Salves and creams can be particularly good for aches and pains associated with aging. Since chronic pain often occurs in elderly patients (especially if there is one localized spot), topical agents can be part of a comprehensive cannabis regiment for elderly patients with localized, chronic pain.

General Recommendations for Using Cannabis and CBD in the Elderly

Different people react differently to medications, including medical cannabis. In addition, especially in older patients, side effects are a concern. Thus, I generally recommend starting with very low doses and slowly increasing the dose to get the desired effect without side effects (dose titration). In addition, since some elderly patients, in particular those with dementia, may not be able to verbalize the beneficial effects of cannabis, or any side effects, adjusting the dose may have to rely entirely on caregiver observation. Thus, using medical cannabis in elderly patients will require patience.

1. **Start with a high-dose CBD capsule or tincture every day.**
   Since CBD may be neuroprotective, can help with anxiety, is anti-inflammatory, may have anticancer properties, and may mitigate some of the side effects of THC, I strongly recommend that all elderly patients start with a daily dose of CBD. I recommend 25 mg to 30 mg of CBD a day in a pill/edible/capsule or tincture. The exception to this dosing is for patients who have decreased appetite, where the dose of CBD should be 15mg of less. CBD can either be a cannabis-derived CBD or pure-hemp-derived CBD, though I generally recommend hemp-derived CBD, as it is less expensive and easier to obtain, and because there is virtually no THC, it will not make you sleepy or high. Also, since there are no psychoactive effects of CBD alone, there is no need to adjust the dose. Patients and/or their caregivers may not see the benefits of CBD for one to two weeks.

2. **Address sleep issues by using nighttime cannabis, including indica-based products with potentially higher doses of THC, and some CBN.**
   Sleep disruption is so common with the elderly, and the lack of a good night's sleep can make multiple conditions worse. Thus, I strongly recommend focusing on sleep first (in addition to taking daily CBD). In fact, CBD plus low-dose nighttime cannabis may

be all that is needed in treating elderly patients. In addition, to THC and CBD, there is also CBN, which stands for cannabinol. Like CBD, CBN is a nonpsychoactive cannabinoid, and CBN is particularly good for sleep. Five milligrams of CBN may be as effective as a 10-mg dose of diazepam (generic for Valium) for inducing sleep. There are both tinctures and edibles that come in 1:1 CBN:THC ratios. Some also contain natural ingredients such as chamomile and melatonin that can be quite effective to help induce sleep. In addition, some tinctures and edibles contain THC from indica strains, and in some states, you can get tinctures as a whole-plant extract of a particular strain.

Since tinctures only take about twenty to thirty minutes to work, and last about four to six hours, an indica-based tincture, especially one containing CBN, is often a great place to start as it can help patients both fall asleep and stay asleep. Start with a ½ dropperful thirty minutes before bedtime, and increase by a ¼ to ½ dropperful each evening until the patient is falling asleep easily and staying asleep. For patients who have more issues staying asleep than falling asleep, a pill or edible may be a better option. While pills or edibles take about an hour to start working, they last six to eight hours. A 5-mg THC edible, particularly if it is an indica strain and/or contains CBN, would be another good option. Start with a half tablet for the first night or two. If that doesn't work, then go up to the one full tablet. You can increase by half a tablet every two nights until the patient is staying asleep.

3. **Use sativa, sativa-predominant hybrid, or balanced hybrid tinctures or edibles two to three times a day to address daytime symptoms such as pain and anxiety.**
   Sativa strains (Sour Diesel, Jack Herer, Green Crack) and sativa-predominant hybrid strains (Blue Dream, Harlequin) tend to work well in elderly patients because they can be uplifting and calming at the same time. Because many symptoms experienced by elderly patients (anxiety, chronic pain) are constantly present, edibles can

be taken a few times a day to control symptoms all day long. Several companies make edibles that contain 5 mg of THC from a sativa strain that can be helpful for elderly patients, and despite having THC, they should not make patients sedated or sleepy. I recommend starting with half a tablet (2.5 mg) two to three times a day, and increase by half a tablet each day/dose to determine the amount that helps with several of the associated symptoms but does not make patients sleepy or high. If a patient is not able to take an edible, then tincture would be the next best step. Some edibles also come in dissolvable form and can be placed under the tongue like a tincture. For tinctures, look carefully at the amount of THC per dose. If this is not indicated on the bottle or packing, you may have to figure out the dose yourself. Total milligrams of THC divided by milliliters per bottle is equal to the dose of one dropperful, and there are usually about twenty drops per dropperful. Similar to the edibles, I would start with 2.5 mg of THC per dose. In certain states, it may be possible to get a specific tincture by strain. In addition to sativa or sativa-predominant hybrids, when both anxiety and pain are issues, balanced hybrids such as ACDC and Cannatonic should be considered.

4. **Use tincture or vape (if possible) on an as-needed basis for more acute symptoms, such as acute pain or severe agitation.** The combination of daily CBD, daytime sativa/sativa-predominant hybrid, and nighttime indica used in either edible or tincture format can alleviate most chronic symptoms that the elderly experience, and thus are an excellent trio of agents for many elderly patients. However, certain conditions can come on suddenly in the elderly, such as acute pain or agitation. If this occurs, something that works more rapidly make be needed. Vape (also known as concentrate) is also likely the best option for acute episodes of pain or agitation. They are also very effective in helping elderly patients fall asleep quickly. Vape has a very rapid onset of action but may not be possible for some elderly patients to use. If patients cannot properly

take a vape, a tincture is the next best thing. In some states, you can get strain-specific tinctures that are whole-plant extracts. Thus, hybrids like Cannatonic or indicas like Northern Lights or Granddaddy Purple may be helpful. In other states, you may only be able to get an indica or hybrid tincture that is not strain specific. There are also a few states that make rapidly dissolving edibles, which have a faster onset of action.

5. **Use topical preparations for localized pain, or in the area of worst pain when multiple areas exist.**
   Topical balms and ointments can be highly effective for elderly patients with localized pain (i.e., pain in once specific area). It can either be used in addition to the regimen above or used exclusively for localized pain. For example, in a patient who only has shoulder pain, especially after activity, a cannabis cream prior to activity may be all that is needed. In contrast, in a patient with severe osteoarthritis in their back, shoulders, hands, but particularly worse in knees can use daily CBD, tinctures, or edibles throughout the day for chronic pain and vape for breakthrough pain (as described above), as well as topical cream on her knees two to three times a day, since this is where pain is the worst.

Chapter 28 Notes

1. Campos, A. C., M. V. Fogaça, A. B. Sonego, and F. S. Guimarães. Cannabidiol, neuroprotection and neuropsychiatric disorders. *Pharmacol Res* 2016 Oct: 112, 119–127.

2. García, C., C. Palomo-Garo, M. García-Arencibia, et al. Symptom-relieving and neuroprotective effects of the phytocannabinoid Δ9-THCV in animal models of Parkinson's disease. *British Journal of Pharmacology* 2011: 163(7), 1495–1506.

3. Xiong, W., C. Tanxing, et al. Cannabinoids suppress inflammatory and neuropathic pain by targeting α3 glycine receptors. *J Exp Med* 2012 Jun 4: 209(6), 1121–1134.

4. Philpott, H. T., M. O'Brien, and J. J. McDougall. Attenuation of early phase inflammation by cannabidiol prevents pain and nerve damage in rat osteoarthritis. *Pain* 2017: 158(12), 2442–-2451.

5. Abuhasira, R., L. B. Schleider, R. Mechoulam, and V. Novack. Epidemiological characteristics, safety and efficacy of medical cannabis in the elderly. *Eur J Intern Med* 2018 Mar: 49, 44–50.

6. Bargnes, V. H., P. B. Hart, S. Gupta, and L. Mechtler. Safety and Efficacy of Medical Cannabis in Elderly Patients: A Retrospective Review in a Neurological Outpatient Setting. American Academy of Neurology (AAN) 2019 Annual Meeting: Abstract P4.1–014. Presented May 8, 2019.

7. Hillen, J. B., Soulsby, N., Alderman, C., and G. E. Caughey. Safety and effectiveness of cannabinoids for the treatment of neuropsychiatric symptoms in dementia: a systematic review. *Therapeutic advances in drug safety* 2019: 10, 1–23.

8. Peprah, K., and S. McCormack. Medical Cannabis for the Treatment of Dementia: A Review of Clinical Effectiveness and Guidelines-CADTH Rapid Response Report: Summary with Critical Appraisal. *Canadian Agency for Drugs and Technologies in Health*, 2019 Jul 17.

9. Shannon, S., et al. Cannabidiol in Anxiety and Sleep: A Large Case Series. *Perm J* 2019: 23, 18–041.

10. Pilgrim, A., and S. Robinson S. An overview of appetite decline in older people. *Nurs Older People* 2015 Jun: 27(5), 29–35.

11. Patel, D., J. Steinberg, and P. Patel. Insomnia in the Elderly: A Review. *J Clin Sleep Med* 2018 Jun 15: 14(6), 1017–1024.

Acknowledgements

There are many people I wish to thank for helping me with this book. In addition to spending many hours researching the literature, I also spoke to many knowledgeable patient care specialists or "bud-tenders" at my local dispensaries for their knowledge and experience. In particular, I would like to thank Andrew Benton from Rise dispensaries and Rabbi James Kahn at Liberty dispensaries. For suggestions regarding the publication of this book, I am grateful to Michael J. Green of M.Revak & Co. for his guidance and expertise. I am indebted to my family for their support, as well as thoughtful suggestions and feedback, including my wife Julie, daughters Allison and Natalie, parents Rina and Sylvan, and sister Debbie and brother-in-law Andrew. Finally, and most importantly, I would like to the thank the many patients I have treated with medical cannabis for helping me gain insights into the best treatments for specific conditions, as well as the encouragement to become an advocate for medical cannabis in order to help others. While there are too many patients to list by name, I wanted to specifically mention Deborah L. Mazia, who was one of the first patients I treated with medical cannabis, and who first suggested that I share this information with others-may her memory be a blessing.

Made in the USA
Las Vegas, NV
08 January 2022

40810861R10192